MKSAP 12
Nephrology

Contributors

Phillip M. Hall, MD, Section Editor*
Director, Renal Function Laboratory
Department of Nephrology and Hypertension
Cleveland Clinic Foundation
Cleveland, OH

Bennett Lorber, MD, FACP, Associate Editor*
Durant Professor of Medicine
Chief, Section of Infectious Diseases
Temple University School of Medicine
Philadelphia, PA

Gerald B. Appel, MD, FACP*
Director Clinical Nephrology
The New York Presbyterian Hospital
Professor of Clinical Medicine
Columbia University College of Physicians and Surgeons
New York, NY

Michael Emmett, MD, MACP*
Chairman of Internal Medicine
Baylor University Medical Center
Dallas, TX

Paul L. Kimmel, MD, FACP*
Professor of Medicine
Division of Renal Diseases and Hypertension
Department of Medicine
George Washington University Medical Center
Washington, DC

Joseph V. Nally Jr., MD*
Department of Nephrology and Hypertension
Cleveland Clinic Foundation
Cleveland, OH

Co-Editors in Chief

Charles J. Hatem, MD*
Associate Professor of Medicine
Harvard Medical School
Cambridge, Massachusetts

William M. Kettyle, MD*
Associate Clinical Professor of Medicine
Harvard Medical School
Cambridge, Massachusetts

Consulting Editor

Ronald A. Arky, MD, MACP*
Charles Davidson Professor of Medicine
Harvard Medical School
Cambridge, Massachusetts

* Has no significant financial relationship with relevant commercial companies/organizations.

Principal Staff

Senior Vice President, Education
Herbert S. Waxman, MD, FACP

Vice President, Education
D. Theresa Kanya, MBA

Director, Self-Assessment Programs
Sean McKinney

Managing Editor
Charles Rossi

Staff Editors for MKSAP 12 Nephrology
Catherine M. Welcher
Charlotte D. Fierman

Production Administrator
Sheila F. O'Steen

Editorial Coordinator
Dale Thuesen

Developed by the American College of Physicians–American Society of Internal Medicine

Acknowledgments

The American College of Physicians–American Society of Internal Medicine (ACP–ASIM) gratefully acknowledges the special contributions to the development and production of the Medical Knowledge Self-Assessment Program® 12 of Valerie Dangovetsky (administrator) and Michael Ripca (graphic designer). Computer scoring and reporting are being done by ACT, the selected test-scoring agency, Iowa City, Iowa. The College also wishes to acknowledge that many other persons, too numerous to mention, have contributed to the production of this book. Without their dedicated efforts, this publication would not have been possible.

Continuing Education

The ACP–ASIM is accredited by the Accreditation Council for Continuing Medical Education to provide continuing medical education for physicians.

The American College of Physicians–American Society of Internal Medicine designates this educational activity for a maximum of 135 hours in Category 1 credit toward the American Medical Association Physician's Recognition Award. Each physician should claim only those hours of credit that he/she actually spent in the educational activity.

Learning Objectives

The learning objectives of the Medical Knowledge Self-Assessment Program are to assess the current state of your medical knowledge, compare your performance on the self-assessment tests with that of your peers, update your knowledge in 13 key areas of internal medicine, apply new clinical problem-solving skills to improve the health of your patients, and pursue further in-depth study using critically reviewed evidence-based references.

In December 1999, the Institute of Medicine (IOM) issued a report challenging the medical profession to work together with hospitals, nurses, the federal government, and other health professions to improve patient safety and reduce avoidable medical errors that may lead to patient injury or death. The ACP–ASIM actively supports the goals of the IOM to improve the quality of patient care and to protect patient safety.

Note

The editors and publisher of Medical Knowledge Self-Assessment Program 12 recognize that the development of new material offers many opportunities for error. Despite our best efforts, some errors may persist into print. Drug dosage schedules are, we believe, accurate and in accordance with current standards. Readers are advised, however, to ensure that the recommended dosages in MKSAP 12 concur with the information provided in the product information material. This is especially important in the case of new, infrequently used, or highly toxic drugs.

Publisher's Information

ISBN: 1-930513-03-8

Library of Congress Catalog Number: 00-105021

Printed in the United States of America.

For order information call 1-800-523-1546, ext. 2600 (in PA call 215-351-2600), or fax inquiries to 215-351-2799.

Table of Contents

Nephrology

Hypertension

An estimated 50 million persons in the United States — about 20% of the adult population and 60% of persons over age 65 — have hypertension. The risk of cardiovascular complications escalates in a continuous, graded, and predictable manner with increases in systemic blood pressure. As evidenced by the Framingham Study and other data, the systolic blood pressure correlates better with cardiovascular risk factors than the diastolic blood pressure.

Table 1 shows the classification of blood pressure according to the Sixth Joint National Committee (JNC-VI) on Detection, Prevention, Evaluation, and Treatment of High Blood Pressure (Sixth report, JNC-VI). Importantly, the authors introduce a new stratification of "normal" blood pressure (< 140/90 mm Hg) to include "optimal," "normal," and "high-normal" blood pressure determinations. The classification of hypertension has been modified to include three stages based upon either systolic or diastolic blood pressure. The authors emphasize that the objective of identifying and treating the hypertensive patient is to control blood pressure and reduce cardiovascular morbidity and mortality.

The sixth report of the Joint National Committee on prevention, detection, evaluation, and treatment of high blood pressure. Arch Intern Med. 1997;157:2413-46. UI: 98046261

The recognition, treatment, and control of hypertension have improved over the last quarter century. Age-adjusted death rates from a stroke have declined by nearly 60% and from coronary artery disease by 53%. However, the recent JNC-VI report offers several sobering notes of caution, as shown in the Key Points.

The JNC-VI report proposes a renewed effort to identify and stage patients with hypertension based on their blood pressure determinations, cardiovascular risk factors, and clinical target organ damage (Table 2). Emphasis will be directed toward therapy for patients who have higher risk with the expectation of achieving greater benefit. For example, a recent analysis reexamined the effect of antihypertensive therapy on mortality rates based on the presence or absence of target organ damage at the time of initiation of therapy for patients with stage 1 hypertension in the Hypertension Detection and Follow-up Program (HDFP) study. Although there was a similar *relative risk* reduction of 22% in both groups, the *absolute* benefit of lives saved per 100 patients treated was greater in the group with target organ damage.

KEY POINTS

- **Hypertension control rates in the United States have not continued to improve.**
- **Only 53% of persons with hypertension are being treated, and only 27% have adequately controlled blood pressure.**
- **Only 45% of patients receiving antihypertensive therapy have a blood pressure < 140/90 mm Hg.**
- **Since 1993, age-adjusted stroke rates have risen slightly, and the rate of decline of coronary artery disease appears to be leveling.**
- **The incidence of end-stage renal disease (for which hypertension is the second most common cause) has increased. Hypertension also contributes to the progression of renal disease in patients with diabetic nephropathy and other glomerular diseases.**
- **The incidence of congestive heart failure (for which the great majority of patients have antecedent hypertension) has increased in the elderly population.**

TABLE 1 Classification of Blood Pressure for Adults Aged 18 Years and Older

Category	Systolic (mm Hg)		Diastolic (mm Hg)	Follow-up
Optimal	< 120	*and*	< 80	–
Normal	< 130	*and*	< 85	Recheck in 2 years
High-normal	130–139	*or*	85–89	Recheck in 1 year
Hypertension				
Stage 1	140–159	*or*	90–99	Confirm in 2 months
Stage 2	160–179	*or*	100–109	Reheck in 1 month
Stage 3	≥ 180	*or*	≥ 110	Immediate follow-up

Adapted from: The sixth report of the Joint National Committee on prevention, detection, evaluation, and treatment of high blood pressure. Arch Intern Med. 1997;157:2413-46.

TABLE 2 Components of Cardiovascular Risk Stratification in Patients with Hypertension

Major Risk Factors	Target Organ Damage/ Clinical Cardiovascular Disease
Smoking	Heart disease
Dyslipidemia	Left ventricular hypertrophy
Diabetes mellitus Age older than 60 years	Angina pectoris/prior myocardial infarction
Gender (men and postmenopausal women)	Prior coronary revascularization
Family history of cardiovascular disease	Heart failure
Women under age 65 *or*	Stroke or transient ischemic attack
Men under age 55	Nephropathy
	Peripheral arterial disease
	Retinopathy

Adapted from: The sixth report of the Joint National Committee on prevention, detection, evaluation and treatment of high blood pressure. Arch Intern Med. 1997;157:2413-46.

Evaluation and Management of the Patient with Hypertension

- What stage of hypertension does a patient with high blood pressure have?
- What is the cardiovascular risk profile of a patient with hypertension?
- What treatment options are appropriate for a patient with hypertension?

Case 1

A 53-year-old woman is evaluated because of "high blood pressure." A series of elevated blood pressure readings averaging 150/95 mm Hg were obtained at her local community center over a 2-month period. The patient has type 2 diabetes mellitus without retinopathy or nephropathy. She also reports a 3-year history of hypertension and a "kidney problem" but denies a history of cardiovascular or renal disease. She is a former smoker and does not use alcohol or recreational drugs. The family history is positive for hypertension and stroke. Her only medication is glyburide, 5 mg daily.

On physical examination, her weight is 60 kg (132 lb). Blood pressure is 148/92 mm Hg both seated and standing. A complete examination and electrocardiogram are normal. Blood urea nitrogen is 18 mg/dL, serum creatinine 1.0 mg/dL, sodium 138 meq/L, potassium 4.0 meq/L, chloride 100 meq/L, and bicarbonate 25 meq/L. Fasting plasma glucose is 158 mg/dL. Plasma cholesterol is 230 mg/dL, triglycerides 280 mg/dL, high-density lipoprotein cholesterol 38 mg/dL, low-density lipoprotein cholesterol 164 mg/dL, and hemoglobin A_{1c} 8%. Serum thyroid-stimulating hormone level and routine urinalysis are normal.

Initial evaluation of the patient with hypertension should include identifying the cause and severity of the hypertension, documenting the presence or absence of target organ damage, and identifying other cardiovascular risk factors.

In Case 1, the patient's clinical presentation, positive family history of hypertension, and normal urinalysis, serum electrolytes, and renal function suggest that primary hypertension is the most likely diagnosis. There is little to suggest the possibility of a secondary cause of hypertension. She has stage 1 hypertension occurring in the setting of diabetes mellitus without overt target organ damage. However, the JNC-VI report equates the presence of diabetes mellitus as being equivalent to the presence of other target organ damage. In contrast to previous reports, the JNC-VI recommends both lifestyle modifications (nonpharmacologic therapy) and drug therapy for a patient with stage 1 hypertension and diabetes mellitus. Current recommendations also suggest a similar approach to patients with diabetes mellitus and "high-normal" blood pressure, given their increased cardiovascular risk factors.

Initial Management of Hypertension

Lifestyle Modifications

These interventions are designed to lower blood pressure and/or reduce cardiovascular risk factors. The most beneficial lifestyle modifications for reducing blood pressure are weight loss, reduction of alcohol intake, a low-salt diet, and exercise. Weight reduction in a patient whose weight is 10% above ideal body weight will lower blood pressure by an average of 5 to 7 mm Hg. Alcohol intake should be limited to two alcoholic beverages a day. Reducing dietary sodium intake has a modest effect on blood pressure, although some patients (such as black Americans and the elderly) may respond dramatically to a low-salt diet. A low-salt diet may also potentiate the effects of some antihypertensive medications (especially diuretics and angiotensin-converting enzyme inhibitors). Regular aerobic physical activity enhances weight loss, reduces cardiovascular risk factors, and minimally lowers blood pressure. Use of potassium supplements and relaxation techniques has had inconsistent effects on reducing blood pressure. Results from randomized clinical trials have failed to establish convincing evidence that calcium, magnesium, fish oil, or garlic supplements are beneficial.

Initiating Pharmacologic Therapy

Effective antihypertensive therapy reduces the likelihood of stroke, coronary events, heart failure, and all-cause mortality; slows progression of renal disease; and prevents the development of more severe hypertension. Several factors should be considered when selecting an initial antihypertensive agent. These include efficacy, side effects, comorbidities, convenience, response, and cost. However, the current evidence, based on randomized, controlled clinical trials, supports the JNC-VI recommendations that diuretics and β-blockers are the preferred initial agents because of their proven efficacy (and perhaps lower cost) in reducing cardiovascular complications.

Thiazide diuretics may be effective in low doses, such as hydrochlorothiazide, 12.5 to 25 mg daily. At these low doses, the metabolic effects (for example, hyperglycemia, hyperuricemia, and hypokalemia) are negligible, and maximal antihypertensive effects can be achieved. *β-Blockers* are well tolerated by many older patients without affecting cognition or mental status. However, β-blockers should be avoided in patients with type 1 diabetes mellitus, asthma, heart block, and depression.

The JNC-VI recommends using angiotensin-converting enzyme (ACE) inhibitors, angiotensin II receptor blockers, calcium channel blockers, α-blockers, and α,β-blockers as alternative initial monotherapy when a diuretic and/or β-blocker is contraindicated or poorly tolerated or when special clinical situations are present. *ACE inhibitors* are especially indicated in treating hypertension in patients with diabetes mellitus, renal disease, and congestive heart failure (see later discussion on Compelling Indications for Antihypertensive

Therapy). ACE inhibitors may cause angioedema, hyperkalemia, and renal failure, and patients should be closely monitored when these agents are first prescribed. *Angiotensin II type 1 receptor blockers (ARBs)* are a new class of agents that pharmacologically block the angiotensin effect at the receptor level. Like ACE inhibitors, ARBs may sustain renal function and can reduce proteinuria. In addition, ARBs do not induce cough and rarely cause angioedema. Whether ARBs will prove to be as effective as ACE inhibitors in improving outcomes in patients with diabetes mellitus, renal disease, and congestive heart failure remains to be proved.

Earlier retrospective studies suggested that the use of *calcium channel blockers* to treat hypertension is associated with an increased risk of myocardial infarction. The apparent adverse effects were confined to short-acting agents that are known to increase sympathetic tone, which, in turn, may increase the risk for cardiovascular events. Although still controversial, most authorities agree that short-acting calcium channel blockers should be avoided in the treatment of hypertension. More recent large prospective clinical trials have not settled the controversy. In the Appropriate Blood Pressure Control in Diabetes (ABCD) trial (Estacio et al.), patients with diabetes mellitus who were randomized to receive dihydropyridine calcium channel blockers had a greater frequency of myocardial infarctions than a cohort who were treated with ACE inhibitors. In contrast, in the multinational Hypertension Optimal Therapy (HOT) trial (Hansson et al.), a long-acting dihydropyridine calcium channel blocker was step 1 therapy for almost 19,000 patients, who had fewer than predicted cardiovascular events. In the Systolic Hypertension in Europe (SYST-EUR) trial (Staessen et al.; Tuomilehto et al.), administration of a dihydropyridine calcium channel blocker reduced the incidence of cardiovascular morbidity and mortality.

For patients with type 2 diabetes mellitus, such as the patient in Case 1, administration of low-dose diuretics appears to be an acceptable choice, as several clinical trials have shown that these agents confer a similar reduction in cardiovascular complications in both diabetic and nondiabetic patients. Antihypertensive drug therapy should be initiated with the goal of reducing blood pressure below 130/85 mm Hg. ACE inhibitors, α-blockers, calcium channel blockers, and low-dose diuretics are preferred because of fewer adverse effects on glucose homeostasis, lipid profiles, and renal function compared with β-blockers and high-dose diuretics. ACE inhibitors may also be first-line therapy because of their known cardioprotective benefits, as shown in the HOPE trial and other studies (Yusuf et al.), and because they prevent microalbuminuria. If a patient has microalbuminuria, ACE inhibitors should be prescribed to reduce the microalbuminuria and preserve renal function. If a patient is unable to tolerate an ACE inhibitor, preliminary studies suggest that an ARB or a non-dihydropyridine calcium channel blocker (diltiazem or verapamil) may have similar renoprotective properties.

Estacio RO, Jeffers BW, Hiatt WR, Biggerstaff SL, Gifford N, Schrier RW. The effect of nisoldipine as compared with enalapril on cardiovascular outcomes in patients with non-insulin-dependent diabetes and hypertension. N Engl J Med. 1998;338:645-52. UI: 98135519

Hansson L, Zanchetti A, Carruthers SG, Dahlof B, Elmfeldt D, Julius S, et al. Effects of intensive blood-pressure lowering and low-dose aspirin in patients with hypertension: principal results of the Hypertension Optimal Treatment (HOT) randomised trial. HOT Study Group. Lancet. 1998; 351:1755-62. UI: 98297870

Staessen JA, Fagard R, Thijs L, Celis H, Arabidze GG, Birkenhager WH, et al. Randomised double-blind comparison of placebo and active treatment for older patients with isolated systolic hypertension. The Systolic Hypertension in Europe (Syst-Eur) Trial Investigators. Lancet. 1997;350:757-64. UI: 97443133

Tuomilehto J, Rastenyte D, Birkenhager WH, Thijs L, Antikainen R, Bulpitt CJ, et al. Effects of calcium-channel blockade in older patients with diabetes and systolic hypertension. Systolic Hypertension in Europe Trial Investigators. N Engl J Med. 1999;340:677-84. UI: 99150065

Yusuf S, Sleight P, Pogue J, Bosch J, Davies R, Dagenais G. Effects of an angiotensin-converting-enzyme inhibitor, ramipril, on cardiovascular events in high-risk patients. The Heart Outcomes Prevention Evaluation Study Investigators. N Engl J Med. 2000;342:145-53. UI: 20092358

Follow-up

The recent JNC-VI report recommends a lower blood pressure target of < 130/85 mm Hg for patients with diabetes mellitus in order to reduce cardiovascular complications of hypertension. Observations from the recent HOT trial, using a cohort of 1500 patients with diabetes mellitus, demonstrated that achieving lower blood pressure targets is associated with fewer myocardial infarctions and cardiovascular events.

If after 1 to 3 months the response to an initial antihypertensive agent is inadequate, the options are: 1) increase the dose of the first drug to maximal levels, if tolerated; 2) add a second agent from another class; or 3) substitute an agent from another class. Combining antihypertensive agents allows lower doses of both drugs to be used, which perhaps minimizes the potential side effects.

Special Clinical Situations in Patients with Hypertension

Secondary Hypertension

Case 2

A 69-year-old male executive is referred to you for evaluation of severe hypertension. Prior to his referral, he had a severe headache and was seen in a local emergency department where his blood pressure was 210/120 mm Hg. He has no history of hypertension, congestive heart failure, stroke, diabetes mellitus, or renal disease. He is a long-term smoker who had a myocardial infarction 2 years ago. Current medications are atenolol and aspirin.

On physical examination, he weighs 70 kg (154 lb). His blood pressure is 216/118 mm Hg seated and standing. Optic fundi show grade II hypertensive changes without hemorrhages, exudate, or papilledema. There is a left carotid bruit. The lungs are clear. Cardiac examination shows a normal sinus rhythm without murmurs or gallops. Abdominal examination is normal except for the presence of a systolic epigastric bruit. Neuromuscular examination is also normal.

Blood urea nitrogen is 20 mg/dL, serum creatinine 1.4 mg/dL, sodium 138 meq/L, potassium 3.3 meq/L, chloride 100 meq/L, and bicarbonate 28 meq/L. Plasma glucose is 96 mg/dL. Plasma cholesterol is 230 mg/dL, and low-density lipoprotein cholesterol is 150 mg/dL. Serum thyroid-stimulating hormone level and urinalysis are normal. An electrocardiogram shows normal sinus rhythm and a remote inferior wall myocardial infarction.

Most patients with secondary hypertension have one of three types: *renal*, *renovascular*, or *endocrine*. Fewer than 10% of patients have secondary forms of hypertension, and most secondary forms can be detected by the history and physical examination (Table 3).

The patient in Case 2 has stage 3 hypertension with clinical target organ damage, as evidenced by his prior myocardial infarction. The presentation of severe hypertension of abrupt onset in an older man with diffuse atherosclerosis obliterans is atypical for primary hypertension and suggests the possibility of a secondary form of hypertension (Table 4). In this patient, the presentation is typical for renovascular hypertension.

TABLE 3 Features Suggesting Secondary Hypertension

Clinical Features
Age of onset < 30 or > 55 years
Abrupt onset, severe hypertension (≥ stage 3)
Hypertension resistant to effective medical therapy
Target organ damage
Fundi with acute hemorrhages or exudates
Renal dysfunction
Left ventricular hypertrophy
Other Features Indicative of Secondary Hypertension
Unprovoked hypokalemia
Abdominal bruit or diffuse atherosclerosis
ACE inhibitor–induced renal dysfunction
Labile hypertension, sweats, tremor, headache
Family history of renal disease
Palpable polycystic kidneys

ACE inhibitor = angiotensin-converting enzyme inhibitor

Renovascular Hypertension

Renovascular hypertension (RVHT) is caused by hemodynamically significant unilateral or bilateral renal artery stenosis and/or obstruction. In more than two thirds of patients, the cause is renal artery atherosclerotic disease. Other less common causes are fibromuscular disease of the renal arteries, arteritis, and arterial dissection. Since RVHT is uncommon, the diagnosis should only be considered in patients with clinical features that are clues to the diagnosis of secondary hypertension (Mann and Pickering).

Mann SJ, Pickering TG. Detection of renovascular hypertension. State of the Art: 1992. Ann Intern Med. 1992;117:845-53. UI: 93036935

TABLE 4 Classification of Hypertension

Type	Prevalence
Essential (primary) hypertension	90%–95%
Secondary hypertension	5%–10%
Renal	2.5%–6.0%
Renal parenchymal disease	
Polycystic kidney disease	
Urinary tract obstruction	
Renin-producing tumor	
Liddle's syndrome	
Renovascular hypertension or renal infarction	0.2%–4.0%
Coarctation of the aorta	—
Endocrine	1%–2%
Oral contraceptives	
Adrenal	
Primary aldosteronism	
Cushing's syndrome	
Pheochromocytoma	
Congenital adrenal hyperplasia	
Hyperthyroidism and hypothyroidism	
Hypercalcemia	
Hyperparathyroidism	
Exogenous hormones – glucocorticoids, mineralocorticoids, sympathomimetics	
Pregnancy-induced hypertension	
Neurogenic	
Alcohol, cocaine, and medications (cyclosporine, erythropoietin)	—

Diagnosis

Since blood pressure control and/or renal function may be improved by surgery or angioplasty with stent placement, diagnostic studies for RVHT should be performed only in patients whose clinical status will permit such therapeutic interventions. It is crucial to remember that not all hypertension in the presence of renal artery stenosis is RVHT. The two conditions may simply coexist. Although renal arteriography is the most accurate procedure for diagnosing RVHT, it does not always detect which patient with renal artery stenosis actually has RVHT. Tests that determine hormonal or hemodynamic consequences of renal artery stenosis are used to identify RVHT and to differentiate it from renal artery stenosis that is not causing hypertension. Determination of random plasma renin activity, intravenous pyelography, and renography without administration of ACE inhibitors will fail to diagnose approximately 25% to 50% of patients with RVHT and are therefore not recommended. Plasma renin activity measured after the administration of ACE inhibitors may have false-negative results in approximately 25% of patients with RVHT. Renal vein renin determination has a sensitivity of 80% but is too invasive and expensive to be a useful screening test. Renography using ^{131}I-hippuran, Tc-DTPA, or Tc-mertiatide (MAG 3) after administration of the oral ACE inhibitor, captopril, can identify RVHT with about 80% sensitivity and specificity, which is comparable to renal vein renin determinations but is a less invasive test. The sensitivity of renography is compromised by the presence of azotemia and bilateral renal artery stenosis. Prospective studies have shown that duplex ultrasonography of the renal arteries has a sensitivity of greater than 90% for both the presence and the degree of renal arterial disease (Olin et al.). However, the accuracy of this study

Olin JW, Piedmonte MR, Young JR, DeAnna S, Grubb M, Childs MB. The utility of duplex ultrasound scanning of the renal arteries for diagnosing significant renal artery stenosis. Ann Intern Med. 1995;122:833-8. UI: 95259937

is operator dependent, and the study is currently not widely available. Magnetic resonance angiography may be used as a noninvasive screening test, but this study is expensive. Three-dimensional images can be obtained by spiral CT; however, this technique requires use of potentially nephrotoxic contrast material.

Management

The hypertension in many patients with RVHT can be well controlled with medical therapy, and adequate renal function can be maintained. Successful correction of renal artery stenosis most often results in cure or amelioration of hypertension in young patients with fibrous renal artery disease and in patients with atherosclerotic renal artery stenosis whose hypertension is of less than 2 years' duration, who have unilateral (rather than bilateral) renal artery stenosis, and who have a positive captopril renogram or lateralizing renal vein renin determinations. In patients with fibromuscular renal artery stenosis, angioplasty has a 60% to 80% success rate for cure or improvement of hypertension and is the preferred treatment method for this disease. Angioplasty will correct the stenosis in only 30% to 50% of patients with atherosclerotic renal artery stenosis and will result in cure or amelioration of hypertension in about 20% to 30% of these patients. Recent reports of renal artery stenting for ostial lesions have claimed excellent initial technical success rates and secondary patency rates of 92% at 27 months of follow-up. However, long-term normalization of blood pressure was achieved in only 16% of patients, and elevated serum creatinine concentrations did not change in patients who had previously impaired renal function. Surgical correction of renal artery stenosis has resulted in cure of hypertension in approximately 61% of patients and amelioration in about 27% of patients with fibromuscular lesions and in cure of hypertension in approximately 38% of patients and amelioration in about 41% of patients with atherosclerotic lesions (Stanley).

Controversy exists regarding management of patients with azotemia and bilateral or unilateral renal artery stenosis. In this clinical setting, it is difficult to predict whether correction of the stenosis will improve renal function and reduce blood pressure, since in many patients both azotemia and hypertension may be caused by renal parenchymal disease. Prospective studies comparing outcomes of surgical versus medical management in this group of high-risk patients are currently being conducted. Recently, three randomized, controlled clinical trials from Europe compared percutaneous transluminal renal angioplasty with medical therapy in patients with atherosclerotic renal artery stenosis (Plouin et al.). Percutaneous transluminal renal angioplasty resulted in only a modest improvement in blood pressure control and medication reduction without a demonstrable improvement in renal function. In addition, the rate of complications was significant. At present, the most appropriate management of patients with atherosclerotic renal artery stenosis is not known (van Jaarsveld et al.; Webster et al.).

In a patient such as the one described in Case 2, duplex ultrasonography or renography with administration of an ACE inhibitor may confirm the clinical suspicion of probable renal artery stenosis. If the patient's blood pressure can be adequately controlled with medication and if renal function is preserved, additional invasive interventions may not be warranted. ACE inhibitors or angiotensin II receptor blockers must be used cautiously for treating such patients because renal dysfunction may occur in the presence of bilateral or unilateral renal artery stenosis. Calcium channel blockers, β-blockers, and diuretics may be suitable alternatives. Providing optimal medical care for patients with atherosclerotic renal artery stenosis includes more than simply managing their hypertension. Modification of cardiovascular risk factors is extremely important

Stanley JC. The evolution of surgery for renovascular occlusive disease. Cardiovasc Surg. 1994;2:195-202. UI: 94326188

Plouin PF, Chatellier G, Darne B, Raynaud A. Blood pressure outcome of angioplasty in atherosclerotic renal artery stenosis: a randomized trial. Essai Multicentrique Medicaments vs Angioplastie (EMMA) Study Group. Hypertension. 1998;31:823-9. UI: 98154655

van Jaarsveld BC, Krijnen P, Pieterman H, Derkx FH, Deinum J, Postma CT, et al. The effect of balloon angioplasty on hypertension in atherosclerotic renal-artery stenosis. Dutch Renal Artery Stenosis Intervention Cooperative Study Group. N Engl J Med. 2000;342:1007-14. UI: 20193152

Webster J, Marshall F, Abdalla M, Dominiczak A, Edwards R, Isles CG, et al. Randomised comparison of percutaneous angioplasty vs continued medical therapy for hypertensive patients with atheromatous renal artery stenosis. Scottish and Newcastle Renal Artery Stenosis Collaborative Group. J Hum Hypertens. 1998;12:329-35. UI: 98318387 because the majority of deaths in these patients are attributable to coronary artery disease and stroke. For example, in the patient in Case 2, careful attention should be given to managing his dyslipidemia, and he should be strongly advised to stop smoking.

Compelling Indications for Antihypertensive Therapy

Using evidence-based medicine from a literature review of clinical trials, the JNC-VI report recommended "compelling indications" for specific classes of antihypertensive agents for management of four disease states that may coexist in the hypertensive patient: isolated systolic hypertension, type 1 diabetes mellitus with proteinuria, heart failure, and post–myocardial infarction (Table 5).

Isolated Systolic Hypertension

Case 3

A 72-year-old retired physician comes to your office for his periodic health assessment. He notes that several blood pressure readings have averaged 175/80 mm Hg in the last 6 to 8 months. Medical history is negative for atherosclerotic heart disease, dyslipidemia, and diabetes mellitus. He is a nonsmoker, uses alcohol only socially, and takes no medications.

On physical examination, his weight is 74 kg (163 lb). His blood pressure is 178/68 mm Hg both seated and standing. Detailed examination is normal. Blood urea nitrogen is 8 mg/dL, serum creatinine 1.0 mg/dL, sodium 140 meq/L, potassium 4.2 meq/L, chloride 103 meq/L, and bicarbonate 24 meq/L. Plasma cholesterol is 212 mg/dL, and urinalysis is normal. An electrocardiogram shows normal sinus rhythm with nonspecific ST-T wave changes.

Hypertension is extremely common in older Americans, affecting approximately 60% of persons over 65 years of age. In elderly patients, systolic blood pressure is a better predictor of cardiovascular events than is diastolic blood pressure. The benefit of therapy for systolic hypertension in persons over 60 years of age has been well-documented in five large, randomized clinical trials.

In the patient in Case 3, the elevated blood pressure may be classified as isolated systolic hypertension (defined as a systolic blood pressure > 140 mm Hg and a diastolic blood pressure < 90 mm Hg) and further categorized as stage 2 hypertension. Elevation of systolic blood pressure even in patients with stage 1 isolated systolic hypertension increases the risk of coronary artery disease, congestive heart failure, cerebrovascular accident, and end-stage renal disease. The benefits of treatment have been demonstrated for patients with

TABLE 5 Compelling Indications for Specific Classes of Antihypertensive Therapy in Concomitant Diseases

Indication	Drug Therapy
Diabetes mellitus with proteinuria	ACE inhibitors
Heart failure	ACE inhibitors, diuretics
Isolated systolic hypertension (older patients)	Diuretics (preferred)
	Long-acting dihydropyridine CCBs
Post–myocardial infarction	β-Blockers
	ACE inhibitors (with systolic dysfunction)

ACE inhibitors = angiotensin-converting enzyme inhibitors; CCBs = calcium channel blockers isolated systolic hypertension with a systolic blood pressure > 160 mm Hg. The benefits of therapy for patients with stage 1 isolated systemic hypertension have not yet been conclusively shown in controlled clinical trials.

Antihypertensive management in older persons should begin with lifestyle modifications, including modest sodium restriction and weight loss (if needed). If target blood pressure is not achieved, pharmacologic therapy should be instituted. The blood pressure goal should be the same as for younger patients (< 140/90 mm Hg), although an interim goal for systolic blood pressure of < 160 mm Hg may be necessary for patients with marked isolated systolic hypertension (Savage et al.). The JNC-VI report recommends low-dose diuretics or dihydropyridine calcium channel blockers as initial therapy for patients with isolated systolic hypertension.

Savage PJ, Pressel SL, Curb JD, Schron EB, Applegate WB, Black HR, et al. Influence of long-term, low-dose, diuretic-based, antihypertensive therapy on glucose, lipid, uric acid, and potassium levels in older men and women with isolated systolic hypertension: The Systolic Hypertension in the Elderly Program. SHEP Cooperative Research Group. Arch Intern Med. 1998;158:741-51. UI: 98213401

In addition to treating isolated systolic hypertension in the elderly, there are "compelling indications" for aggressive and specific antihypertensive treatment for three other disease states: type 1 diabetes mellitus with proteinuria, heart failure, and post–myocardial infarction.

Type 1 Diabetes Mellitus with Proteinuria

In patients with type 1 diabetic nephropathy, ACE inhibitors have demonstrated an impressive renoprotective effect in slowing the progression of diabetic renal disease. A similar renoprotective effect has been noted in patients with nondiabetic renal disease. A more detailed discussion of specific antihypertensive therapy and lower target blood pressure goals for patients with proteinuric renal disease is provided in the later section on Chronic Renal Insufficiency. In these patients, the blood pressure goal is < 130/85 mm Hg (or < 125/75 mm Hg in patients with urinary protein > 1 g/24 h).

Heart Failure

The Framingham Study has demonstrated that hypertension continues to be the major risk factor for left ventricular hypertrophy, myocardial ischemia, and congestive heart failure. Evidence from clinical trials has shown that most antihypertensive agents, especially ACE inhibitors, are effective in either preventing or causing regression of left ventricular hypertrophy. Since ACE inhibitors are effective in reducing morbidity and mortality in patients with congestive heart failure, patients with both hypertension and congestive heart failure will benefit from these drugs. When ACE inhibitors are contraindicated or are not tolerated, the vasodilator combination of hydralazine and nitrates is also effective in these patients. In addition, the α,β-blocker, carvedilol, has also proved to be beneficial. A trial with the angiotensin II receptor blocker, losartan, for patients with congestive heart failure has provided encouraging data (Pitt et al.). Two dihydropyridine calcium channel blockers, amlodipine and felodipine, have been shown to be safe in treating angina pectoris in patients with hypertension and advanced left ventricular dysfunction. Other calcium channel blockers are not recommended for such patients.

Pitt B, Poole-Wilson PA, Segal R, Martinez FA, Dickstein K, Camm AJ, et al. Effect of losartan compared with captopril on mortality in patients with symptomatic heart failure: randomised trial - the Losartan Heart Failure Survival Study ELITE II. Lancet. 2000;355:1582-7. UI 20279381

Post–Myocardial Infarction

Patients with hypertension and known coronary artery disease are at high risk for cardiovascular morbidity and mortality. The benefits and safety of antihypertensive therapy for such patients have been well documented. The JNC-VI report recommends a target blood pressure of < 140/90 mm Hg for these patients. Furthermore, results of the HOT trial suggest that diastolic blood pressure may be safely lowered to approximately 80 mm Hg even in the subset of patients with ischemic heart disease. However, excessively rapid lowering of

KEY POINTS

- The JNC-VI report introduced a new stratification of blood pressure measurements to include:
  - Optimal (< 120/80 mm Hg)
  - Normal (< 130/85 mm Hg)
  - High normal (130–139/85–89 mm Hg)
- During the initial evaluation, the physician should identify and stage patients with hypertension based on their blood pressure determinations, cardiovascular risk factors (especially diabetes mellitus), and presence or absence of clinical target organ damage.
- For secondary forms of hypertension, the physician should think: renal, renovascular, and endocrine diseases.
- Lower target blood pressure goals are recommended in two select populations:
  - Patients with diabetes mellitus (blood pressure < 130/85 mm Hg)
  - Patients with renal disease (blood pressure < 130/85 mm Hg [< 125/75 mm Hg if urinary protein is > 1 g/24 h])

systemic blood pressure should be avoided, especially when such rapid reduction causes reflex tachycardia and sympathetic activation.

In patients who have sustained a myocardial infarction, there are "compelling indications" for administration of β-blockers without intrinsic sympathomimetic activity because these agents reduce the risk of subsequent myocardial infarction or sudden cardiac death. If β-blockers are contraindicated or are not tolerated, verapamil or diltiazem may be used. ACE inhibitors are also useful after myocardial infarction in patients with left ventricular systolic dysfunction.

Clinical Evaluation of Renal Function

- What are the most important considerations in using the serum creatinine measurement as an estimate of the glomerular filtration rate?
- How does one assess the importance of urinary dipstick proteinuria?

The presence and extent of parenchymal renal disease are usually detected by abnormalities in serum creatinine or creatinine clearance; by a urinalysis showing proteinuria, pyuria, or hematuria; or by abnormalities on renal imaging studies.

Serum Creatinine/Creatinine Clearance

Case 4

A 20-year-old healthy muscular male college athlete weighing 94 kg (206 lb) and a 68-year-old woman with hypertension weighing 55 kg (120 lb) are in your office on the same day. The college student needs a physical examination for a summer job, and the woman is being seen for a routine health maintenance visit. In each, the urinalysis shows 1+ protein, and the serum creatinine is 1.4 mg/dL.

Walser M. Assessing renal function from creatinine measurements in adults with chronic renal failure. Am J Kidney Dis. 1998;32:23-31. UI: 98332083

Measurement of serum creatinine concentration is the most frequently used test to assess functional renal mass (Walser). The serum creatinine level in any individual is the result of 1) the endogenous production of creatinine, which correlates with muscle mass and tends to be constant in the same individual, and 2) the renal excretion of creatinine by glomerular filtration and, to a lesser extent, by proximal tubular secretion. The latter increases with worsening renal insufficiency and decreases with administration of drugs such as cimetidine and trimethoprim. The influence of muscle mass and tubular secretion of creatinine on the serum creatinine concentration is illustrated by the following points. A serum creatinine level of 1.0 mg/dL may represent a normal glomerular filtration rate (GFR) in a healthy man with a normal muscle mass but may represent a GFR of 40% to 60% of normal in an elderly woman with a smaller muscle mass. Studies comparing the serum creatinine level with the measured GFR have shown that at a serum creatinine of 1.1 mg/dL, 10% of men and 50% of women have an abnormal GFR; at a serum creatinine of 1.5 mg/dL, 50% of men and 90% of women have an abnormal GFR. In Case 4, although the serum creatinine concentration in these two individuals is the same, the renal function will be significantly different. The young muscular man will likely have normal renal function, whereas the elderly woman will likely have renal function at 50% to 60% of normal.

In general, individuals who are elderly, chronically ill, and of female gender have smaller muscle mass and hence a lower serum creatinine concentration at any level of GFR (Table 6). At all levels of GFR, black men and women have a

TABLE 6 Serum Creatinine:GFR Relationships

Males		Females	
Serum Cr (mg/dL)	**GFR (% Abn)**	**Serum Cr (mg/dL)**	**GFR (% Abn)**
1.1	10%	0.7	10%
1.5	50%	1.1	50%
1.8	90%	1.6	90%

Abn = abnormal; Cr = creatinine; GFR = glomerular filtration rate

higher serum creatinine concentration than do their white counterparts (Levey et al.). Several additional caveats are important in understanding the clinical use of serum creatinine concentration to estimate GFR. In patients with slowly progressive renal failure, a rise in the serum creatinine level may underestimate the real change in GFR because of the increased tubular secretion of creatinine that occurs as azotemia worsens. Conversely, an increase in serum creatinine of 0.3 to 1.0 mg/dL may occur without any actual change in GFR because of inhibition of tubular secretion of creatinine by cimetidine or trimethoprim. Ketone bodies, cephalosporins, methanol, and isopropyl alcohol interfere with the Jaffe reaction used to measure serum creatinine, resulting in a spuriously elevated value.

To more accurately estimate functioning renal mass, the creatinine clearance must be determined. Because of tubular secretion of creatinine, creatinine clearance often overestimates the true GFR by 20% to 40% in patients with mild to moderate azotemia. Figure 1 shows the relationships between serum creatinine, muscle mass, creatinine clearance, and true GFR. Numerically small increases in serum creatinine concentration are associated with fairly significant reductions in GFR when the functioning nephron mass is reduced from normal to about 50% of normal. The Cockcroft-Gault formula [serum creatinine = (140 – age) × weight in kg/72 × (creatinine clearance in mg/dL)], which may

Levey AS, Bosch JP, Lewis JB, Greene T, Rogers N, Roth D. A more accurate method to estimate glomerular filtration rate from serum creatinine: a new prediction equation. Modification of Diet in Renal Disease Study Group. Ann Intern Med. 1999;130:461-70. UI: 99165393

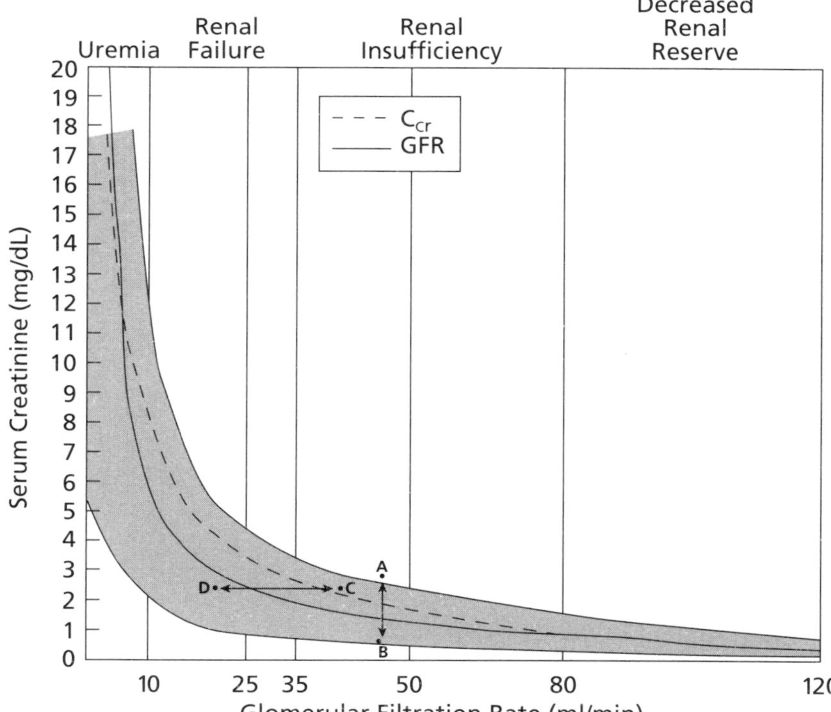

FIGURE 1
The relationship between the serum creatinine (Scr), muscle mass (shaded area), glomerular filtration rate (GFR), and creatinine clearance (Ccr) in patients with normal renal function and in those with renal insufficiency, renal failure, and uremia. The solid line represents the relationship between Scr and GFR as measured by ^{125}I-iothalamate urinary clearance. The dashed line represents the relationship between Scr and Ccr. At any particular GFR level, the width of the shaded area shows the range of Scr that might be seen as a result of differences in muscle mass. Points A and B show the differing levels of Scr in two patients having high (A) or low (B) muscle mass but the same GFR. Points C and D show the same Scr in two patients having a significantly different GFR. The Ccr most significantly overestimates the GFR in the range of renal function designated "Renal Insufficiency" and "Renal Failure," where the Scr is most difficult to use as an estimate of functioning renal mass.

Zaltzman JS, Whiteside C, Cattran DC, Lopez FM, Logan AG. Accurate measurement of impaired glomerular filtration using single-dose oral cimetidine. Am J Kidney Dis. 1996;27:504-11. UI: 96272313

be used to estimate creatinine clearance, includes corrections for age and body size (muscle mass). The correlation between this formula method and actual GFR measurements is reasonably good except in patients at the extremes of age and body size and in patients with acute renal failure in whom the serum creatinine level is changing rapidly. Creatinine clearance measured after administering 800 mg of oral cimetidine also correlates well with actual GFR (Zaltzman et al.). When more precise GFR measurements are needed, various isotopic urinary clearance methods, such as the clearance of ^{125}I-iothalamate, can be used. Although these methods are safe and accurate, they are rarely used in routine clinical situations.

Urinalysis

Proteinuria

Larson, TS. Evaluation of proteinuria. Mayo Clin Proc. 1994;69:1154-8. UI: 95057345

In Case 4, understanding the significance of the dipstick proteinuria requires several considerations. Urinary protein is easily detected by the colorimetric dipstick method, which depends on proteins, especially albumin, causing a color change in the indicator dye (Larson). This method detects concentrations of protein as low as 15 mg/dL. Thus, normal amounts of protein may cause a positive reaction in a concentrated urine specimen; conversely, significant proteinuria may not be detected in very dilute urine. In addition, false-positive reactions for protein may occur in highly alkaline urine and in urine contaminated with certain antiseptics (such as benzalkonium chloride and chlorhexidine). Since albumin is primarily detected by the dipstick method, renal diseases associated with immunoglobulins or light chains in the urine (myeloma or plasma cell dyscrasias) may cause a negative dipstick reaction and can only be detected by turbidimetric methods such as use of sulfosalicylic acid. Transient dipstick proteinuria (a trace or 1+ dipstick reaction for protein that may be associated with fever or exercise) is rarely of clinical significance. In Case 4, the most important first consideration is to verify whether the dipstick proteinuria is persistent. If so, urine sediment should be examined, and, when indicated, a 24-hour urinary protein measurement should be obtained.

The renal diseases causing persistent qualitative proteinuria can be further categorized by quantifying 24-hour protein excretion. Normally, the daily urinary excretion of protein is less than 100 mg. Of this, 60% is derived from filtered plasma proteins (10 to 30 mg of which is albumin), and 40% consists of tissue proteins (some of which are secreted by the uroepithelial cells). A 24-hour urine collection for protein is commonly used to quantify the degree of proteinuria. Alternatively, a spot urine specimen for protein and creatinine concentrations in mg/dL will provide a protein:creatinine ratio that compares well with the 24-hour protein quantification. With this method, a protein:creatinine ratio of 0.1 is equivalent to a normal daily protein excretion of 100 mg or less, and a protein:creatinine ratio of 3 or more is associated with a daily protein excretion of greater than 3 g (an amount consistent with nephrotic-range proteinuria).

Proteinuria may result from conditions that cause 1) "overflow" proteinuria, which is due to elevated normal or abnormal plasma proteins (monoclonal proteins, light chains); 2) increased glomerular permeability, which occurs in various forms of glomerulonephritis in which the proteinuria frequently exceeds 2 to 3 g/24 h; 3) decreased reabsorption of normally filtered plasma proteins, which occurs in patients with tubulointerstitial disease and usually causes proteinuria of less than 2 g/24 h; and 4) an alteration in renal hemodynamics, which seems to explain the mild degrees of proteinuria that occur with fever, physical exercise, standing upright, major motor seizures, and other conditions associated with stimulation of the renin-angiotensin system and reduction in renal plasma flow. This last type of proteinuria is frequently transient and benign.

Microalbuminuria refers to the excretion of albumin in the range of 30 to 300 mg/24 h (15 to 200 µg/min). Quantitative measurement of albumin excretion cannot be done by the usual dipstick or qualitative protein methods. Instead, sensitive immunoassay techniques are needed. In normal persons, urinary albumin excretion is < 30 mg/24 h. Screening for microalbuminuria is done by measuring the albumin:creatinine ratio in a first-voided morning urine specimen or by using highly sensitive dipsticks (Bennett et al.). Testing for microalbuminuria may be of greatest clinical value in detecting the earliest stages of diabetic nephropathy. Heavy exercise, urinary tract infection, acute febrile illnesses, and heart failure may transiently increase microalbuminuria. Because nonsteroidal anti-inflammatory drugs and angiotensin-converting enzyme (ACE) inhibitors can decrease urinary protein excretion, screening for microalbuminuria should be done when these drugs are not being administered.

Bennett PH, Haffner S, Kasiske BL, Keane WF, Mogensen CE, Parving HH, et al. Screening and management of microalbuminuria in patients with diabetes mellitus: Recomendations to the Scientific Advisory Board of the National Kidney Foundation from the ad hoc committee of the Council on Diabetes Mellitus of the National Kidney Foundation. Am J Kidney Dis. 1995; 25:107-12. UI: 95109520

Hematuria

Hematuria is defined by the presence of > 3 to 5 erythrocytes per high-power field (hpf). Hematuria is most easily detected by using the dipstick strip, which is impregnated with orthotolidine. This is sensitive enough to detect > 5 erythrocytes/hpf. A positive dipstick reaction for blood is also caused by urine containing free hemoglobin and myoglobin, urine containing ascorbic acid exceeding 5 mg/dL, or urine contaminated by the antiseptic povidone iodine (Betadine). A urine sample that is dipstick positive for blood but has no erythrocytes on microscopic examination suggests a false-positive reaction caused by myoglobin, povidone iodine, or ascorbic acid (due to ingestion of vitamin C) or may result from lysis of erythrocytes in a dilute urine specimen (specific gravity usually < 1.006). Isolated hematuria commonly occurs in women during menstruation; in patients with urologic diseases, such as neoplasms of the urogenital tract, nephrolithiasis, and renal cystic disease; and in patients with hematologic disorders, such as coagulopathies and sickle cell disease. The hematuria accompanying most glomerular diseases is associated with significant proteinuria; the finding of erythrocyte casts or dysmorphic erythrocytes is indicative of glomerular disease as well.

KEY POINT

- Diagnostic clues to causes of isolated hematuria include:
  - Menstruation
  - Urologic neoplasms
  - Renal cystic disease
  - Coagulopathies
  - Sickle cell disease
  - Nephrolithiasis

Leukocyturia

Normally, the urine contains < 3 to 5 leukocytes/hpf. If clean voiding techniques are carefully followed, the number of leukocytes in the urine is the same for both men and women. Polymorphonuclear leukocytes contain esterases. Reagent dipstick strips detect leukocytes by the action of these esterases, which causes a color change in 1 to 2 minutes. The dipstick method is able to detect leukocytes in excess of 3 to 4 leukocytes/hpf with a sensitivity of 92%. Leukocyturia frequently occurs in patients with urinary tract infections but may also occur in patients with tubulointerstitial disease and in some patients with renal stones even in the absence of infection.

Renal Imaging Techniques

Although abdominal radiographs can visualize the kidneys, measure renal size, and show calcifications in the urogenital tract, they are rarely used as the initial imaging technique in evaluating renal disease. Spiral CT without contrast is frequently used in the initial evaluation of patients with renal stone disease because all stones will be visualized by this modality.

Renal Ultrasonography

Renal ultrasonography has become the initial imaging technique used in the evaluation of renal disease because it can be performed at any level of renal function, is noninvasive, and requires no potentially nephrotoxic contrast material. Renal ultrasonography accurately measures renal size, readily detects obstruction, and has excellent resolution for evaluating renal masses and differentiating them from renal cysts. A solid mass must usually exceed 3 cm in size to be readily detected by ultrasonography. Staging of renal masses is better done with CT. Both radiopaque and radiolucent renal stones may be detected by ultrasonography, although stones smaller than 5 mm may be missed. Prospective studies have shown that duplex ultrasonography of the renal arteries has a sensitivity of greater than 90% for identifying both the presence and the degree of renal artery disease (Olin et al.). This technique is noninvasive, but the accuracy is operator dependent. Visualization of the renal arteries may be hindered by body habitus, bowel liquid or gas, and movement of the patient.

Olin JW, Piedmonte MR, Young JR, DeAnna S, Grubb M, Childs MB. The utility of duplex ultrasound scanning of the renal arteries for diagnosing significant renal artery stenosis. Ann Intern Med. 1995;122:833-8. UI: 95259937

Intravenous Pyelography

Intravenous pyelography is done following bolus injection of an iodinated radiocontrast agent. However, it carries the risk of nephrotoxicity, especially in patients with diabetes mellitus and azotemia. Intravenous pyelography is still used to evaluate patients with nonglomerular hematuria, renal stones, urinary tract infections, voiding disorders, and unexplained flank or abdominal pain. It is not a sensitive or specific technique for diagnosing renovascular disease or predicting the likelihood of interventional cure of renovascular hypertension.

Computed Tomography

CT of the kidneys relies on tissue density differences to distinguish anatomic structures. Spiral CT without contrast is reserved for investigation of renal calculus disease or for evaluation of suspected renal or perirenal hemorrhage. Iodinated-contrast–enhanced CT allows better definition of renal masses. Simple benign renal cysts have an imperceptibly thin wall, are homogeneous and of the same density as water, create a distinct interface with the renal parenchyma, and do not enhance with intravenous contrast agents. Renal neoplasms distort the renal contour, do not have a sharp interface with the surrounding renal parenchyma, are heterogeneous, and enhance with intravenous contrast agents. CT is also helpful for diagnosing angiomyolipomas and for staging of renal neoplasms, which may be bilateral or multifocal or may have spread into the renal veins, the inferior vena cava, or the periaortic and retroperitoneal lymph nodes.

Radionuclide Scans

The radionuclide scan is primarily used to assess renal perfusion and is especially useful for detecting significant differences in perfusion between the kidneys. Severe or complete reduction in renal perfusion is easily detected with this technique, especially when involvement is unilateral. The renogram has a 75% sensitivity for detecting hemodynamically significant renal artery stenosis. Sensitivity is increased to 92% by repeating the renogram after administration of oral captopril.

Renal Arteriography

Renal arteriography is used primarily to assess renal artery disease. Risks associated with arteriography include atheroembolic and contrast-mediated acute renal failure. MRI can be used to identify renal vein thrombosis. MRI is becoming increasingly useful in the evaluation of renal artery disease, and in some institutions the quality of MRI is close to that of arteriography.

Renal Biopsy

Renal biopsy is performed primarily to diagnose glomerular disease or unusual causes of acute renal failure. It is usually performed with ultrasound or CT guidance and should only be done by those who have had experience with the procedure and its risks. Uncontrolled hypertension, bleeding disorders, active urinary tract infection, and a solitary kidney are relative contraindications to percutaneous needle biopsy of the kidney. Complications include perinephric bleeding or small arteriovenous fistulae following almost all biopsies. About 1 in 10 patients has gross hematuria, 1 in 100 patients requires a blood transfusion, and 1 in 1000 patients requires nephrectomy. When a biopsy is necessary in a high-risk patient, a laparoscopic or transjugular approach may be appropriate.

Glomerular Diseases

Glomerular diseases affect millions of persons worldwide and are significant causes of end-stage renal disease. Although similar mechanisms may underlie the manifestations of glomerular disease (such as hematuria, erythrocyte casts, proteinuria), different processes may initiate this damage. Immune-mediated renal injury is a major pathogenetic mechanism of glomerular damage. Different mechanisms are involved in other diseases, such as amyloidosis.

The Nephrotic Syndrome

- What are the common manifestations of the nephrotic syndrome and the potential mechanisms that produce them?
- How are the clinical manifestations of the nephrotic syndrome treated?
- What are common causes of primary and secondary nephrotic syndrome?
- What diagnostic tests help distinguish the various forms of the nephrotic syndrome?
- Which types of therapy are available to treat the specific forms of the nephrotic syndrome?

Case 5

A previously healthy 36-year-old black American man is evaluated because of periorbital edema in the morning and swelling of his ankles and feet in the evening. He has gained 10 kg (22 lb) in 2 weeks. On physical examination, his blood pressure is 140/88 mm Hg. The remainder of the examination is normal except for pedal edema. Blood urea nitrogen is 14 mg/dL, serum creatinine is 1.1 mg/dL, and serum electrolytes are normal. Plasma glucose is 102 mg/dL. Plasma cholesterol is 387 mg/dL. Serum albumin is 2.2 g/dL, serum complement is normal, and the antinuclear antibody titer is negative. Urinalysis shows 4+ protein with occasional erythrocytes and oval fat bodies. Urinary protein excretion is 11g/24 h.

This patient has the nephrotic syndrome, which is defined as a urinary albumin concentration > 3.0 to 3.5 g/24 h accompanied by hypoalbuminemia, edema, and hyperlipidemia (Orth and Ritz). Hypoalbuminemia results from urinary protein loss as well as from catabolism of filtered albumin by the proximal tubules and redistribution of albumin within the body. The nephrotic edema in this patient may be due to two different mechanisms: 1) proteinuria leading to hypoalbuminemia, a low plasma oncotic pressure, and intravascular volume depletion with stimulation of the renin-angiotensin-aldosterone axis causing

Orth SR, Ritz E. The nephrotic syndrome. N Engl J Med. 1998;338:1202-11. UI: 98209526

KEY POINTS

- The nephrotic syndrome is defined by significant albuminuria. If urinary albumin is < 3.0 to 3.5 g/24 h, the patient does not have the nephrotic syndrome regardless of other clinical findings.
- Edema, hyperlipidemia, and a procoagulant tendency are all common manifestations of the nephrotic syndrome. Each can be treated effectively even if the underlying glomerular disease is not cured.
- Membranous nephropathy is the most common cause of idiopathic nephrotic syndrome in adult Americans, but focal segmental glomerulosclerosis is more common among black Americans.

Maschio G, Alberti D, Janin G, Locatelli F, Mann JF, Motolese M, et al. Effect of the angiotensin-converting-enzyme inhibitor benazepril on the progression of chronic renal insufficiency. The Angiotensin-Converting-Enzyme Inhibition in Progressive Renal Insufficiency Study Group. N Engl J Med. 1996;334:939-45. UI: 96175229

Ponticelli C, Passerini P. Treatment of nephrotic syndrome associated with primary glomerulonephritis. Kidney Int. 1994;46:595-604. UI: 95089273

sodium retention, or 2) primary renal sodium retention at a distal nephron site, perhaps due to altered responsiveness to atrial natriuretic factor. Most patients with the nephrotic syndrome have elevated levels of total and low-density lipoprotein cholesterol and lipoprotein(a). These patients have an increased risk for atherosclerotic complications, perhaps in part related to their hyperlipidemia. Some patients, especially those patients with marked proteinuria and hypoalbuminemia, have a procoagulant tendency and may develop deep venous thrombosis or pulmonary emboli. The causes of this clotting tendency are multifactorial and include increased platelet aggregation, increased fibrinogen concentration, and loss of anti-clotting factors such as antithrombin III in association with the proteinuria.

The use of angiotensin-converting enzyme (ACE) inhibitors and angiotensin II receptor blockers in patients with the nephrotic syndrome has been associated with decreased proteinuria, hypoalbuminemia, and hyperlipidemia (Maschio et al.). This patient's edema can be treated with a low-salt diet and potent loop diuretics. His hyperlipidemia can be managed with a low-cholesterol, low-saturated-fat diet and use of lipid-lowering medications such as 3-hydroxy-3-methylglutaryl–coenzyme A (HMG-CoA) reductase inhibitors. He may be given an ACE inhibitor or an angiotensin II receptor blocker to reduce his proteinuria. Since he does not have diabetes mellitus and his serologic studies are nondiagnostic, he is likely to have idiopathic nephrotic syndrome. Although many different serologic tests may be needed to evaluate a patient with the nephrotic syndrome, almost all patients should have an antinuclear antibody titer to screen for collagen disease and a serum complement determination to exclude the forms of glomerulonephritis listed in Table 7 that are associated with hypocomplementemia. The treatment and course of patients with idiopathic nephrotic syndrome depend on the specific histologic pattern found at renal biopsy (Ponticelli and Passerini) (Table 8).

Minimal Change Disease

The histologic pattern of minimal change disease may be found in from 10% to 15% of adults with the idiopathic nephrotic syndrome. Minimal change disease may also occur in association with use of nonsteroidal anti-inflammatory drugs and lithium and in patients with Hodgkin's disease and leukemia. Almost all patients present with edema, and adults may have hypertension, microhematuria, and even moderate azotemia related to hypoalbuminemia and volume depletion. Some elderly patients with minimal change disease develop acute reversible renal failure that may respond to diuresis. Light microscopy shows no glomerular abnormalities, and immunofluorescence staining and electron microscopy show no immune deposits. Electron microscopy does show effacement of visceral epithelial foot processes along virtually all capillary loops, which is a correlate of the significant albuminuria.

The course of patients with minimal change disease is often one of remissions and relapses. Treatment with high-dose glucocorticoids usually leads to remission of proteinuria. Adults are not considered glucocorticoid-resistant until they have failed to respond to 16 weeks of therapy. At least 30% to 50% of patients will relapse within 1 year. Retreatment with glucocorticoids often leads to further remissions. In patients who have frequent relapses or patients who are glucocorticoid-dependent, treatment with an oral alkylating agent (such as cyclophosphamide or chlorambucil) often leads to a prolonged remission of the nephrotic syndrome. Cyclosporine may be used as an alternative agent, but carries a risk of nephrotoxicity and a higher relapse rate.

TABLE 7 Nephrotic Syndrome Associated with Specific Causes (Secondary Nephrotic Syndrome)

Systemic Diseases

Diabetes mellitus*

Systemic lupus erythematosus* and other collagen diseases

Amyloidosis (associated with AL amyloid or AA amyloid)

Vasculitic-immunologic diseases (mixed cryoglobulinemia, Wegener's granulomatosis, rapidly progressive glomerulonephritis, polyarteritis, Henoch-Schönlein purpura, sarcoidosis, Goodpasture's syndrome)

Infections

Bacterial (poststreptococcal, congenital and secondary syphilis, subacute and acute bacterial endocarditis, shunt nephritis)

Viral (hepatitis B,* hepatitis C,* HIV,* infectious mononucleosis)

Parasitic (malaria, toxoplasmosis, schistosomiasis, filariasis)

Medication-related

Nonsteroidal anti-inflammatory drugs*

Gold, mercury, and heavy metals

Penicillamine

Lithium

Paramethadione, trimethadione

"Street" heroin

Others — probenecid, chlorpropamide, rifampin, tolbutamide, phenindione

Allergens, Venoms, and Vaccines

Associated with Neoplasms

Hodgkin's lymphoma and leukemia-lymphomas (with minimal change lesions)

Solid tumors (with membranous nephropathy)

Hereditary and Metabolic Diseases

Alport's syndrome

Fabry's disease

Sickle cell disease

Congenital (Finnish-type) nephrotic syndrome

Familial nephrotic syndrome

Nail-patella syndrome

Partial lipodystrophy

Others

Pregnancy-related (includes preeclampsia)

Transplant rejection

Serum sickness

Accelerated hypertensive nephrosclerosis

Unilateral renal artery stenosis

Massive obesity-sleep apnea

Reflux nephropathy

*Most common disorders.

TABLE 8 Causes of Primary Nephrotic Syndrome

Idiopathic or Primary Nephrotic Syndrome	Incidence*
Minimal change disease	10% to 15%
Focal segmental glomerulosclerosis	20% to 25%
Membranous nephropathy	25% to 30%
Membranoproliferative glomerulonephritis	5%
Other forms of glomerulonephritis	15% to 30%

*In adult Americans.

Focal Segmental Glomerulosclerosis

Focal segmental glomerulosclerosis (FSGS) is the most common form of idiopathic nephrotic syndrome in black Americans. It may also be secondary to heroin use, HIV infection, sickle cell disease, obesity, urinary reflux, or the presence of a solitary kidney with reduced function. The patient in Case 5, an adult black American with idiopathic nephrotic syndrome, is likely to have FSGS. At presentation, about 66% of patients with FSGS are nephrotic, and approximately 30% to 40% have hypertension, microscopic hematuria, and a decreased glomerular filtration rate (GFR).

Renal biopsy shows glomerulosclerosis in part of the glomerular tuft of only some glomeruli, but electron microscopy demonstrates effacement of foot processes in all glomerular capillaries, which is indicative of the generalized increased permeability to albumin (Savin et al.). As renal function declines, repeat biopsies show more segmental areas of glomerulosclerosis, more globally scarred glomeruli, and secondary interstitial scarring. Spontaneous remission of proteinuria is uncommon, and patients without remission typically develop end-stage renal disease in 5 to 10 years. Patients who are nephrotic and have greater degrees of proteinuria and those with interstitial scarring on biopsy are most likely to develop renal failure.

Savin VJ, Sharma R, Sharma M, McCarthy ET, Swan SK, Ellis E, et al. Circulating factor associated with increased glomerular permeability to albumin in recurrent focal segmental glomerulosclerosis. N Engl J Med. 1996;334:878-83. UI: 96175826

Appel GB. Focal segmental glomerulosclerosis. In: Greenberg A, ed. Primer on Kidney Disease. San Diego: Academic Press; 1998:160-4. UI: 9717616

Treatment of FSGS is controversial, and there are few randomized, controlled clinical trials. However, studies using more intensive and longer courses (6 to 12 months) of glucocorticoids and other immunosuppressive agents have reported a 40% to 60% remission rate of the nephrotic syndrome with preservation of long-term renal function. A randomized, blinded clinical trial of use of cyclosporine in patients with glucocorticoid-resistant FSGS has shown that this agent is beneficial in inducing remission of proteinuria and preservation of the GFR (Appel).

Membranous Nephropathy

Membranous nephropathy is the most frequent cause of idiopathic nephrotic syndrome in adult Americans. It may also be associated with infections (such as syphilis and hepatitis B), systemic lupus erythematosus, certain medications (such as gold salts), and certain solid tumors and lymphomas. Patients present with edema, often associated with hypertension and microhematuria. The GFR is often normal at presentation. Membranous nephropathy is the most common form of the nephrotic syndrome associated with thrombotic events, including renal vein thrombosis. Renal vein thrombosis may be asymptomatic, may be associated with a decreased GFR and increased proteinuria in the nephrotic patient, or may present as pulmonary emboli. Histologic renal specimens in patients with membranous nephropathy show thickened glomerular capillary loops without cellular proliferation. Immunofluorescence studies show immunoglobulins and complement in a fine granular distribution along the glomerular capillary walls, and electron microscopy reveals subepithelial electron-dense deposits.

Both the slow progression and the spontaneous remission rate of membranous nephropathy have confounded clinical treatment trials. Survival with adequate renal function is usually greater than 75% at 10 years, and the spontaneous remission rate is 20% to 30%. The results of retrospective and prospective controlled clinical trials have not clearly defined whether short courses of glucocorticoids increase the remission rate of proteinuria or preserve long-term renal function. Several recent controlled clinical trials have reported a greater number of total remissions and better preservation of renal function when using either cytotoxic agents alternating with monthly glucocorticoids or glucocorticoids alone for 6 months (Hogan et al.; Ponticelli et al.). Other studies have

Hogan SL, Muller KE, Jennette JC, Falk RJ. A review of therapeutic studies of idiopathic membranous glomerulopathy. Am J Kidney Dis. 1995;25:862-75. UI: 95289400

Ponticelli C, Zucchelli P, Passerini P, Cesana B, Locatelli F, Pasquali S, et al. A 10-year follow-up of a randomized study with methylprednisolone and chlorambucil in membranous nephropathy. Kidney Int. 1995;48:1600-4. UI: 96130553

concluded that treatment results are no better than the natural history of the disease (Schieppati et al.). Patients who are older, who are male, who had reduced renal function prior to developing membranous nephropathy, and especially those who have greater degrees of persistent heavy proteinuria are at greatest risk for developing progressive disease. These patients are most likely to benefit from immunosuppressive therapies.

Schieppati A, Mosconi L, Perna A, Mecca G, Bertani T, Garattini S, et al. Prognosis of untreated patients with idiopathic membranous nephropathy. N Engl J Med. 1993;329:85-9. UI: 93288086

Johnson RJ, Gretch DR, Couser WG, Alpers CE, Wilson J, Chung M, et al. Hepatitis C virus-associated glomerulonephritis. Effect of alpha-interferon therapy. Kidney Int. 1994;46:1700-4. UI: 95214407

Membranoproliferative Glomerulonephritis

Membranoproliferative glomerulonephritis (MPGN) is an uncommon form of idiopathic nephrotic syndrome. Many patients who were formerly thought to have an idiopathic disorder are now known to have renal disease associated with hepatitis C virus infection or systemic lupus erythematosus (Johnson et al.). Although most patients with MPGN have the nephrotic syndrome, some present with microhematuria and proteinuria or with an acute nephritic syndrome. A low serum complement level is found intermittently in patients with type I MPGN, whereas serum C3 levels are always reduced in patients with type II MPGN. Although no therapy has been proved effective in adults, a large, randomized, controlled clinical trial has shown that children given long-term alternate-day glucocorticoids had greater remissions of the nephrotic syndrome and preservation of renal function.

AL Amyloidosis

AL amyloidosis is a systemic disease caused by the overproduction of monoclonal immunoglobulin light chains (80% of which are lambda chains). Up to 80% of patients with this disorder have renal involvement, most often albuminuria, the nephrotic syndrome, and renal insufficiency. Diagnosis may be made from gingival, rectal, fat pad, or renal biopsy. Amyloid appears as amorphous, eosinophilic, extracellular deposits in the glomeruli, along the tubules, and in the renal vessels. AL amyloid is Congo red–positive and appears as extracellular nonbranching 8- to 10-nm fibrils on electron microscopy. Many patients with amyloidosis develop renal failure in 1 to 2 years.

Melphalan and prednisone chemotherapy directed at the abnormal clone of B cells has been shown to benefit some patients (Kyle et al.). Secondary renal amyloidosis is associated with serum amyloid A protein deposition. Therapy should be directed towards correcting the inflammatory condition underlying the production of the amyloid. In some patients, colchicine has led to remission of the nephrotic syndrome and stabilization of renal dysfunction.

Kyle RA, Gertz MA, Greipp PR, Witzig TE, Lust JA, Lacy MQ, et al. A trial of three regimens for primary amyloidosis: colchicine alone, melphalan and prednisone, and melphalan, prednisone, and colchicine. N Engl J Med. 1997;336:1202-7. UI: 97244527

Light-chain Deposition Disease

Light-chain deposition disease is a systemic disorder caused by the overproduction and extracellular deposition of monoclonal light chains. However, it is not associated with the Congo red–staining properties and extracellular nonbranching fibrils characteristic of AL amyloidosis. Most patients have proteinuria, often leading to the nephrotic syndrome and accompanied by hypertension and renal insufficiency. Renal biopsy shows eosinophilic granular glomerular nodules. Immunofluorescence studies demonstrate a single class of immunoglobulin light chains (kappa chains in 80% of patients) along glomerular and tubular basement membranes. Chemotherapy, similar to that for patients with AL amyloidosis, may lead to prolonged renal function and patient survival.

HIV Nephropathy

Patients infected with HIV may develop several types of glomerular damage, including HIV nephropathy (D'Agati and Appel). This usually occurs in black

D'Agati V, Appel GB. HIV infection and the kidney. J Am Soc Nephrol. 1997; 8:138-52. UI: 97165698

patients and most commonly develops at a later stage of HIV infection, when the viral load is high but not necessarily when the patient has an opportunistic infection. HIV nephropathy is characterized by heavy proteinuria, large echogenic kidneys on ultrasonography, and rapid progression to renal failure. The pathologic findings of HIV nephropathy, although resembling findings of FSGS, differ from the findings of heroin nephropathy and classic FSGS. HIV nephropathy is characterized by diffuse glomerular collapse and sclerosing glomerulopathy with severe tubulointerstitial damage and microcystic dilatation of the tubules.

The use of immunosuppressive agents to alter the course of HIV nephropathy is controversial. However, both ACE inhibitors and antiviral agents are standard drugs that are used to try to reduce proteinuria and delay progression of the disease.

Cryoglobulinemia

Mixed cryoglobulinemia is due to the production of circulating immunoglobulins that precipitate ex vivo upon cooling. It is associated with infections, collagen-vascular disease, and lymphoproliferative disorders. Many patients with membranoproliferative glomerulonephritis and cryoglobulinemia who were originally thought to have idiopathic disease have been found to have renal disease associated with hepatitis C. Most patients have proteinuria and slow deterioration of renal function. Hypocomplementemia, especially of the early complement components Clq–C4, is a characteristic finding. Interferon plus ribavirin may reduce proteinuria and improve the GFR in patients with hepatitis C–related cryoglobulinemia, but relapses frequently occur when these medications are stopped.

Acute Glomerulonephritis

- What are the common manifestations of acute glomerulonephritis?
- What diseases are associated with acute glomerulonephritis, and what diagnostic tests distinguish them from one another?
- What treatments are available for the various types of acute glomerular diseases?

Case 6

A previously healthy 55-year-old woman develops malaise, low-grade fever, cough, and shortness of breath. She has a 3-month history of relapsing bronchitis and sinus infections treated with antibiotics. Over the last week, she has developed ankle edema and decreasing urine output.

On physical examination, she appears fatigued and chronically ill. Her temperature is 37.8 °C (100.8 °F). Her pulse rate is 92/min, respiratory rate is 18/min, and blood pressure is 170/100 mm Hg. The maxillary sinuses are tender, and there is no light reflex on her right tympanic membrane. Breath sounds are decreased in the left lower lung field, and crackles are audible. Cardiac examination is normal. There is mild pedal edema. Hematocrit is 29%, the leukocyte count is 16,400/µL, and the platelet count is 428,000/µL. Blood urea nitrogen is 62 mg/dL, serum creatinine is 3.6 mg/dL, and serum electrolytes and plasma glucose are normal. The erythrocyte sedimentation rate is 88 mm/h, serum complement is normal, and the antinuclear antibody titer is negative. Antineutrophil cytoplasmic antibody (ANCA) titers: cytoplasmic ANCA (C-ANCA) positive (1:160); perinuclear ANCA (P-ANCA) negative.

Urinalysis shows 4+ heme and 2+ protein with many dysmorphic erythrocytes and erythrocyte casts on microscopic examination. Chest radiograph shows a left lower lobe infiltrate with cavitation, and sinus films show clouding of the right and left maxillary sinuses.

This patient has acute glomerulonephritis with a nephritic syndrome characterized by a decreased GFR, oliguria, hypertension, and a urine sediment with erythrocytes and erythrocyte casts. Although most patients with acute forms of glomerulonephritis have some proteinuria, most do not have nephrotic-range proteinuria. Renal biopsy shows glomerular hypercellularity due to infiltrating inflammatory cells, proliferation of resident glomerular cells, or both, which can damage the glomeruli by mediators such as oxidants, chemoattractants, proteases, cytokines, and growth factors.

IgA Nephropathy

The most common form of idiopathic glomerulonephritis worldwide is IgA nephropathy. Characteristic presenting findings are asymptomatic microscopic hematuria with or without proteinuria, or, especially in young adults, episodic gross hematuria following upper respiratory tract infections or exercise. Mesangial proliferation is commonly found on light microscopy. The diagnosis is established by the finding of glomerular IgA deposits on immunofluorescence studies. The antibody is usually polymeric IgA_1, which originates in the secretory-mucosal system. However, the antigen (whether viral, dietary, or other) to which the antibody is directed is unknown.

The course of IgA nephropathy is variable. Some patients show no decline in GFR over decades and others develop increased proteinuria, hypertension, and renal failure. Survival of renal function is estimated to be 85% to 90% at 10 years and 75% to 80% at 20 years. Serum IgA levels do not correlate with the course of the disease. Most attempts to treat IgA nephropathy by preventing antigenic stimulation, including use of broad-spectrum antibiotics and dietary manipulations, have been unsuccessful. The benefit of immunosuppressive agents remains unclear. At least one randomized, controlled clinical trial has shown an improved GFR in patients with IgA nephropathy who were treated with fish oils (Donadio et al.). However, smaller studies have provided conflicting results.

Donadio JV Jr, Bergstralh EJ, Offord KP, Spencer DC, Holley KE. A controlled trial of fish oil in IgA nephropathy. Mayo Nephrology Collaborative Group. N Engl J Med. 1994;331:1194-9. UI: 95021562

Henoch-Schönlein Purpura

Henoch-Schönlein purpura is characterized by arthralgias, purpura, and abdominal symptoms along with the renal findings of microscopic hematuria, mild proteinuria, and variable degrees of azotemia. Renal biopsy shows a proliferative glomerulonephritis with IgA immune deposits. There is no proven therapy, and most symptoms resolve spontaneously. Patients with severe glomerulonephritis may benefit from immunosuppressive therapy or from intravenous gamma globulin (as reported in a recent clinical trial), but these treatments are unproved.

Poststreptococcal Glomerulonephritis

Patients with acute poststreptococcal glomerulonephritis (PSGN) may present with an acute nephritic syndrome or with isolated hematuria and proteinuria. PSGN occurs following a latency period of 10 days to several weeks after infection with nephritogenic strains of group A β-hemolytic streptococci. Most patients develop antibodies against streptococcal antigens (including antistreptolysin O, antihyaluronidase, antistreptokinase, and anti-DNAse) and have a change in titer indicative of recent infection. The serum total complement level and C3 level are decreased in more than 90% of patients during the acute episode. Because the serum complement concentration is decreased in only a few types of glomerular disease, it is a useful test for differentiating various forms of glomerulonephritis (Table 9). Because the patient in Case 6 has a normal serum complement level, she is unlikely to have PSGN, systemic lupus erythematosus, cryoglobulinemia, or idiopathic membranoproliferative glomerulonephritis.

PSGN is an immune-complex disease during its acute phase, which is characterized by formation of antibodies against streptococcal antigens and deposition of immune complexes and complement in the kidney. The glomeruli are markedly enlarged and hypercellular, and electron microscopy shows scattered, large, dome-shaped, immune-type subepithelial deposits. The disease is usually self-limited, and renal function recovers in several weeks. Proteinuria and hematuria resolve more slowly.

Immune-complex Glomerulonephritis

Other infections may be associated with acute glomerulonephritis. Proliferative immune-complex glomerulonephritis occurs more commonly in patients with acute rather than subacute bacterial endocarditis and is especially common in patients with staphylococcal endocarditis. Patients often have a nephritic syndrome and reduced serum total complement and C3 levels. A similar immune-complex glomerulonephritis may occur in patients with deep visceral bacterial abscesses, empyema, severe pneumonia, osteomyelitis, and certain viral infections.

Rapidly Progressive Glomerulonephritis

Rapidly progressive glomerulonephritis (RPGN) is a disorder that progresses to renal failure in weeks to months. Renal biopsy shows extensive crescent formation (an extracapillary proliferation). The presentation is of acute nephritis with oliguria, hypertension, edema, and urinary sediment filled with erythrocytes and erythrocyte casts. Different types of RPGN are classified by their immune pathogenesis (Table 10) as being associated with anti–glomerular basement membrane (anti-GBM) antibodies, with immune-complex deposition, or without immune-complex deposits on immunofluorescence studies or electron microscopy. The prognosis has dramatically improved recently for many patients with RPGN.

In anti-GBM disease, circulating antibodies directed against the alpha 3 chain of type 4 collagen can damage the GBM and lead to a proliferative crescentic glomerulonephritis. Linear deposition of immunoglobulin occurs along the GBM. Anti-GBM antibodies that cross-react with the basement membranes

TABLE 9 Serum Complement Levels in Glomerular Diseases

Diseases Associated with a Reduced Serum Complement Level
Postinfectious glomerulonephritis (poststreptococcal glomerulonephritis, subacute bacterial endocarditis, visceral abscesses)
Systemic lupus erythematosus
Cryoglobulinemia
Idiopathic membranoproliferative glomerulonephritis
Diseases Associated with a Normal Serum Complement Level
Minimal change nephrotic syndrome, focal segmental glomerulosclerosis, membranous nephropathy
IgA nephropathy, Henoch-Schönlein purpura
Anti–glomerular basement membrane disease
Pauci-immune rapidly progressive glomerulonephritis, polyarteritis nodosa, Wegener's granulomatosis

TABLE 10 Classification of Rapidly Progressive (Crescentic) Glomerulonephritis

Primary

Anti–glomerular basement membrane antibody disease (with pulmonary disease, Goodpasture's syndrome)

Immune complex–mediated glomerulonephritis

Pauci-immune glomerulonephritis [usually antineutrophil cytoplasmic antibody (ANCA)-positive]

Secondary

Membranoproliferative glomerulonephritis

IgA nephropathy, Henoch-Schönlein purpura

Poststreptococcal glomerulonephritis

Systemic lupus erythematosus

Polyarteritis nodosa, hypersensitivity angiitis

of pulmonary capillaries may cause pulmonary hemorrhage in association with the glomerulonephritis (Goodpasture's syndrome). Intensive therapy with immunosuppressive agents to reduce the production of anti-GBM antibodies and with plasmapheresis to remove circulating anti-GBM antibodies may be beneficial in patients who have not already developed severe renal failure.

Both primary glomerulopathies (for example, IgA nephropathy and idiopathic membranoproliferative glomerulonephritis) and diseases of known etiology (for example, postinfectious glomerulonephritis and systemic lupus erythematosus) may be associated with a crescentic immune-complex glomerulonephritis. The course and therapy of RPGN associated with immune-complex deposition depend upon the type of disease.

Pauci-immune RPGN (without immune-complex deposits) may present as isolated glomerulonephritis with progressive renal failure and a nephritic syndrome or may be associated with systemic vasculitis. Most patients have antineutrophil cytoplasmic antibodies (ANCA) directed against components of neutrophil primary granules. P-ANCA is usually directed against granulocyte myeloperoxidase, whereas C-ANCA is directed against a granulocyte serine proteinase. Patients with positive P-ANCA titers may have clinical features of polyarteritis, whereas patients with positive C-ANCA titers often have extrarenal granulomatous disease, such as Wegener's granulomatosis. There is considerable overlap between groups. The patient in Case 6 has a clinical picture consistent with Wegener's granulomatosis with sinus and lower respiratory tract disease, acute nephritis with oliguria, hypertension, edema, abnormal urinary sediment, and a positive C-ANCA titer. Although patients with various autoimmune and other diseases may have "false-positive" P-ANCA titers, C-ANCA positivity is usually associated with true vasculitis and glomerulonephritis, as in the patient in Case 6. Renal biopsy is likely to show a pauci-immune RPGN. The value of following ANCA levels to monitor the course of patients who have RPGN without immune-complex deposition is controversial (De'Oliviera et al.). Administration of oral or intravenous cyclophosphamide along with glucocorticoid therapy has led to markedly improved patient survival and survival of renal function (Hoffman et al.; Nachman et al.).

De'Oliviera J, Gaskin G, Dash A, Rees AJ, Pusey CD. Relationship between disease activity and anti-neutrophil cytoplasmic antibody concentration in long-term management of systemic vasculitis. Am J Kidney Dis. 1995;25:380-9. UI: 95177162

Hoffman GS, Kerr GS, Leavitt RY, Hallahan CW, Lebovics RS, Travis WD, et al. Wegener granulomatosis: an analysis of 158 patients. Ann Intern Med. 1992; 116:488-98. UI: 92152591

Nachman PH, Hogan SL, Jennette JC, Falk RJ. Treatment response and relapse in antineutrophil cytoplasmic autoantibody-associated microscopic polyangiitis and glomerulonephritis. J Am Soc Nephrol. 1996;7:23-32. UI: 96403829

Lupus Nephritis

Patients with systemic lupus erythematosus (SLE) can present with findings of acute glomerulonephritis, with the nephrotic syndrome, and, rarely, with asymptomatic urinary findings. Although clinical renal disease is variable, histologic involvement is found in renal biopsies from almost all patients with SLE.

The World Health Organization (WHO) classification of lupus nephritis is a useful guide to prognosis and therapy (Table 11). Patients with normal biopsies by light microscopy or those with mesangial proliferation (WHO classes I and II) usually have only mild proteinuria, microscopic hematuria, and preserved renal function and do not require therapy for their renal disease. Patients with mild focal proliferative disease (WHO class III) may present with similar clinical features as classes I and II and also often have a benign renal prognosis. Patients with more severe focal glomerulonephritis will have more proteinuria, hypertension, and abnormal urinary sediment and may have the nephrotic syndrome. Renal biopsy often shows active necrotizing lesions and large amounts of subendothelial deposits similar to findings in patients with active diffuse proliferative disease (WHO class IV). Positive serologic studies for SLE and a nephritic or nephrotic syndrome are all common in patients with diffuse proliferative lupus nephritis. Patients with membranous SLE (WHO class V) often have severe proteinuria and the nephrotic syndrome but have less serologic SLE activity.

Clinical trials in patients with severe lupus nephritis have shown that cyclophosphamide is superior to glucocorticoids for preserving renal function. Patients treated with oral or intravenous cyclophosphamide (every-third-month high doses, for example, 1 g/m^2) or combinations of oral azathioprine and cyclophosphamide have fewer episodes of renal failure at 10 and 20 years than those treated initially with high-dose glucocorticoids or azathioprine alone. Plasmapheresis has not been of added benefit when a regimen of cytotoxic agents and glucocorticoids is used. Recent studies have demonstrated that six consecutive monthly doses of intravenous cyclophosphamide are more effective than pulse intravenous glucocorticoids and that follow-up intravenous cyclophosphamide every third month after the initial 6 months results in fewer episodes of lupus nephritis and renal failure. Although combined therapy with monthly intravenous cyclophosphamide and glucocorticoids is more effective than either agent alone, the combined regimen has the greatest incidence of side effects (Appel and Valeri; Austin et al.; Gourley et al.).

Appel, GB, Valeri A. The course and treatment of lupus nephritis. Annu Rev Med. 1994;45:525-37. UI: 94256789

Austin HA 3rd, Boumpas DT, Vaughan EM, Balow JE. Predicting renal outcomes in severe lupus nephritis: contributions of clinical and histologic data. Kidney Int. 1994;45:544-50. UI: 94217376

Gourley MF, Austin HA 3rd, Scott D, Yarboro CH, Vaughan EM, Muir J, et al. Methylprednisolone and cyclophosphamide, alone or in combination, in patients with lupus nephritis. A randomized, controlled trial. Ann Intern Med. 1996;125:549-57. UI: 96389179

TABLE 11 World Health Organization Classification of Lupus Nephritis

	Class	Clinical Findings
I.	Normal glomeruli (LM, IF, EM)	No renal findings
II.	Mesangial disease	Mild clinical renal disease; minimally active urinary sediment; mild to moderate proteinuria (never nephrotic syndrome) but may have active SLE serology
III.	Focal proliferative glomerulonephritis	More active urinary sediment; often active SLE serology; increased proteinuria (about 25% nephrotic syndrome); hypertension may be present; may evolve into a class IV pattern
IV.	Diffuse proliferative glomerulonephritis	Most severe renal involvement with active urinary sediment, hypertension, heavy proteinuria (frequent nephrotic syndrome), often reduced GFR; SLE serology very active
V.	Membranous glomerulonephritis	Significant proteinuria (often nephrotic syndrome) with less active SLE serology

EM = electron microscopy; GFR = glomerular filtration rate; IF = immunofluorescence; LM = light microscopy; SLE = systemic lupus erythematosus

Renal Microthromboses

Thrombotic microangiopathies, hemolytic-uremic syndrome (HUS), thrombotic thrombocytopenic purpura (TTP), the antiphospholipid syndrome, and the use of drugs such as mitomycin, cyclosporine, and tacrolimus have been associated with microthromboses of the glomerular capillaries and small arterioles. The renal findings may be overshadowed by the systemic features of the microangiopathy. Renal manifestations include gross or microscopic hematuria, proteinuria, renal insufficiency, and oliguric or nonoliguric acute renal failure. Antiplatelet therapy and treatment with glucocorticoids have been effective in some patients with TTP/HUS. Plasma infusion and plasmapheresis may also lead to major improvement in some patients with TTP/HUS, including those with infectious complications. Approximately 40% to 75% of patients with SLE produce antiphospholipid autoantibodies, including anticardiolipin antibodies and/or the lupus anticoagulant, which ironically is associated with thrombotic events. Some patients have thrombotic microangiopathy with evidence of coagulation in their glomeruli and arterioles, whereas others may develop renal vein thrombosis. Patients who have experienced thrombotic events may benefit from high-dose warfarin anticoagulation.

Asymptomatic Urinary Abnormalities

- What findings on urinalysis should prompt further evaluation for a form of glomerular damage?
- What types of glomerular disease commonly present with asymptomatic urinary findings, and how should they be followed and treated?

Case 7

A 38-year-old white man is evaluated because of 4+ hematuria and trace proteinuria detected during an insurance physical examination. Medical history and physical examination, including blood pressure, are normal. Repeat urinalysis again shows 4+ heme and 1+ protein. Microscopic examination shows many erythrocytes, some of which are dysmorphic. No erythrocyte casts are found. Complete blood count, serum electrolytes, and plasma glucose are normal. Blood urea nitrogen is 14 mg/dL, and serum creatinine is 0.8 mg/dL. Serum total complement is normal, and the antinuclear antibody titer is negative.

This patient has asymptomatic microhematuria and proteinuria, which may be due to the early phase of progressive glomerular disease or to a benign glomerular lesion. The dysmorphic erythrocytes on urinalysis point to a glomerular origin for his hematuria (as would the presence of erythrocyte casts). Such patients often have IgA nephropathy. Some patients have familial nephritis or thin–basement membrane disease, a usually benign glomerulopathy associated with areas of focal thinning of the glomerular basement membrane. In general, a renal biopsy is not indicated for patients with urinary protein of < 1 g/24 h, a normal GFR, and no evidence of systemic disease. These patients should be followed for evidence of increasing proteinuria or declining renal function (increasing blood urea nitrogen and serum creatinine levels), at which time renal biopsy should be done.

Tubulointerstitial Diseases

- What are the clinical and urinary manifestations of tubulointerstitial diseases?
- What diseases cause predominantly tubulointerstitial damage to the kidney?
- What diagnostic tests should be done in the evaluation of patients with tubulointerstitial disease?

Tubulointerstitial Nephritis

Case 8

A 32-year-old woman with a long history of chronic headaches is evaluated because of intermittent left colicky flank pain. She denies taking any medications. On physical examination, she is anxious and in moderate distress and is holding her left side. She is afebrile. Her pulse rate is 94/min, respiratory rate is 18/min, and blood pressure is 140/88 mm Hg. Examination of the heart and lungs is normal. Her abdomen is soft with normal bowel sounds, and she has mild left costovertebral angle tenderness.

Blood urea nitrogen is 28 mg/dL, serum creatinine 1.8 mg/dL, sodium 140 meq/L, potassium 4.2 meq/L, chloride 112 meq/L, and bicarbonate 20 meq/L. Plasma glucose is normal. Arterial blood gas studies (with the patient breathing room air) are pH 7.32, Pco_2 32 mm Hg, Po_2 96 mm Hg, and bicarbonate 20 meq/L. Urinalysis shows microhematuria without dysmorphic erythrocytes or erythrocyte casts and no proteinuria.

The patient is treated with narcotics and hydration for presumed acute nephrolithiasis. Renal ultrasonography shows slightly small echogenic kidneys without stones. CT scan of the kidneys shows evidence of papillary necrosis. Repeat discussion with the patient reveals a long history of excessive use of analgesics, including over-the-counter nonsteroidal anti-inflammatory drugs.

Tubulointerstitial nephritis predominantly affects the tubules and the interstitial space between the tubules, rather than the glomeruli and renal vasculature. The disorder may be acute or chronic and may cause structural and functional changes that may be reversible or permanent. Most patients with tubulointerstitial nephritis do not have biopsy documentation of the renal lesion, and the diagnosis is made on clinical grounds and history taking. As does the patient in Case 8, patients with tubulointerstitial nephritis often have hyperchloremic metabolic acidosis due to impaired ammoniagenesis and a bland urinary sediment without heavy proteinuria, dysmorphic erythrocytes, or erythrocyte casts. Some patients also have evidence of papillary necrosis.

Allergic interstitial nephritis, which is an acute and reversible form of tubulointerstitial nephritis, is discussed in the later section on Acute Renal Failure.

The use of medications, including analgesic combinations with phenacetin, acetaminophen, and aspirin; nonsteroidal anti-inflammatory drugs; lithium; the chemotherapeutic agents cisplatin, methyl-CCNU (lomustine), and BCNU (carmustine); and the immunosuppressive agents cyclosporine and tacrolimus may be associated with the development of slow, insidious chronic renal insufficiency and chronic interstitial nephritis.

The prevalence of analgesic nephropathy varies greatly according to the geographic area. In the United States, it accounts for 1% to 10% of patients with end-stage renal disease. In addition, some patients with end-stage renal disease of "unknown etiology" probably actually have analgesic nephropathy as the cause of their renal failure. The reason why the causative analgesic or drug combination induces renal damage is unclear. Retrospective case-controlled studies confirm the finding of significantly more renal disease in persons who use analgesics (Elseviers and De Broe). The risk of renal disease is increased with daily use of phenacetin or acetaminophen but not with aspirin. The classic patient with analgesic nephropathy has chronic headaches or arthritis and has taken large amounts of the causative drugs over many years (as did the patient in Case 8). Renal findings include nocturia and polyuria, sterile pyuria, a predisposition to volume depletion, renal colic, hematuria, and hypertension. Papillary necrosis is often found on CT or on intravenous pyelography. Renal insufficiency is often progressive if analgesic use is continued. Chronic use of nonsteroidal anti-inflammatory drugs may produce an identical clinical and histopathologic picture (De Broe and Elseviers; Henrich et al.).

Elseviers MM, De Broe ME. A long-term prospective controlled study of analgesic abuse in Belgium. Kidney Int. 1995; 48:1912-9. UI: 96163252

De Broe ME, Elseviers MM. Analgesic nephropathy. N Engl J Med. 1998; 338:446-52. UI: 98117073

Henrich WL, Agodoa LE, Barrett B, Bennett WM, Blantz RC, Buckalew VM Jr, et al. Analgesics and the kidney: summary and recommendations to the Scientific Advisory Board of the National Kidney Foundation from an Ad Hoc Committee of the National Kidney Foundation. Am J Kidney Dis. 1996;27:162-5. UI: 96132385

A review of almost 500 patients who required chronic lithium therapy showed that only 15% to 17% of patients had a reduced glomerular filtration rate (GFR) and that the reduction was usually mild. However, this percentage may increase as more patients are being exposed to prolonged use of lithium. The role of other psychotropic medications in causing renal dysfunction remains to be clarified.

Cyclosporine and tacrolimus may cause both acute renal damage and chronic tubulointerstitial fibrosis. Microvascular damage to the renal arterioles may occur, and a chronic form of tubulointerstitial damage in a band-like pattern, called "striped fibrosis," may develop.

Cholesterol Emboli

Atheromatous cholesterol emboli may cause both acute and chronic renal insufficiency. The emboli may occur spontaneously or after angiographic or vascular surgical procedures. Symptoms and signs include fever, livedo reticularis, petechial lesions, retinal vessel occlusions, and digital ischemia. Leukocytosis, transient eosinophilia, hypocomplementemia, and an elevated erythrocyte sedimentation rate may also be present. Most patients are hypertensive and have developed progressive renal insufficiency over weeks to months. The diagnosis is confirmed by biopsy of muscle, skin, kidney, or other organs. Biopsy specimens show typical biconcave clefts in small vessels. There is no effective treatment. Management consists of control of hypertension and supportive therapy.

Reflux Nephropathy, Urinary Tract Infections, and Pyelonephritis

Back flow of urine from the bladder into the upper urinary tract (vesicoureteral reflux) can cause chronic tubulointerstitial damage. Whether sterile reflux without associated infection causes renal damage is unclear. In animals, extravasated sterile refluxed Tamm-Horsfall protein may cause an autoimmune inflammatory response and renal damage. Focal segmental glomerulosclerosis, perhaps due to hyperfiltration of remnant nephrons, may develop in patients with severe reflux. Low-grade reflux may be treated with long-term antibiotic therapy to prevent renal infection. Surgical intervention does not usually prevent progressive renal insufficiency in adults. Patients who have a urinary protein of

> 1.5 g/24 h, a very depressed GFR, and significant renal scarring often develop renal failure.

Episodes of acute bacterial pyelonephritis in a patient with renal obstruction or urinary reflux may lead to chronic pyelonephritis. Chronic pyelonephritis may present insidiously with renal insufficiency associated with hypertension, salt wasting, a urinary concentrating defect, and hyperkalemia. The kidneys are small with asymmetric cortical scars. Xanthogranulomatous pyelonephritis is a localized chronic bacterial renal infection with granuloma formation and lipid-laden macrophages. It usually develops in patients with obstructed kidneys that often contain stones. CT and MRI may help establish the diagnosis. Treatment consists of antibiotic therapy and surgical resection of the abscessed area.

Toxic and metabolic interstitial nephritis may be caused by disorders of calcium oxalate, uric acid, and potassium. Exposure to lead and cadmium may also cause tubulointerstitial nephritis. Precipitation of calcium oxalate can cause nephrolithiasis and tubulointerstitial damage with intratubular and interstitial crystals surrounded by inflammation and fibrosis. Patients with primary hyperoxaluria have a recessive genetic disorder with enzymatic defects in the metabolism of glyoxylic acid and excessive urinary excretion of oxalate. In addition, calcium oxalate may precipitate in the kidneys. By 20 years of age, patients with this disorder may develop end-stage renal disease as a result of infection or obstruction. Oxalate-induced renal damage may also occur following ingestion of ethylene glycol, use of methoxyflurane, excessive intake of ascorbic acid, or excessive intestinal absorption of oxalate in patients with steatorrhea. The treatment of oxalate-induced renal damage includes correction of the primary defect, a low-oxalate diet, increased intake of fluids, and use of pyridoxine (vitamin B_6) supplements.

Hyperuricosuria and urate deposition can cause acute oliguric renal failure associated with myeloproliferative disorders and tumor lysis syndromes. Recent studies suggest that when patients with gout or chronic asymptomatic hyperuricemia develop chronic tubulointerstitial damage, the damage is due to concurrent hypertension, ischemia, and diabetic changes. Hypercalcemia and calcium salt deposition in the tubules and interstitium are associated with chronic interstitial inflammation, fibrosis, and nephrocalcinosis. Patients may have a decreased GFR, polyuria, and nocturia.

Lead may also accumulate in the proximal tubules. The source of the lead may be from pica, alcoholic beverages stored in lead crystal containers or contaminated with lead during production ("moonshine whiskey"), exposure to lead batteries, or industrial aerosolized ingestion. The accumulated lead may cause tubular defects such as Fanconi's syndrome, aminoaciduria, potassium excretory defects, and renal glycosuria as well as renal insufficiency, hypertension, and gout due to disordered renal processing of uric acid (saturnine gout). Serum lead levels are typically normal, and the diagnosis is made by demonstrating excessive urinary excretion of chelated lead after an injection of ethylenediaminetetraacetic acid (EDTA). Renal biopsy will show chronic tubulointerstitial nephritis. Cadmium, which is used in metallurgy, can also cause chronic tubulointerstitial nephritis with tubular defects.

Winearls CG. Acute myeloma kidney. Kidney Int. 1995;48:1347-61. UI: 96099771

Renal involvement is common in patients with multiple myeloma (Winearls). Most patients present with isolated proteinuria. Clinical clues suggesting a diagnosis of myeloma-induced renal disease include 1) little proteinuria on urinary dipstick testing but heavy proteinuria on 24-hour quantification (the dipstick test is far more sensitive to albumin than to globulins); 2) a low anion gap (due to the cationic charge contributed by the abnormal immunoglobulin); 3) hypercalcemia in the presence of renal failure and a high serum phosphorus level; and 4) anemia disproportionate to the degree of renal insufficiency. Renal insufficiency is present in greater than 50% of patients and correlates with patient survival. Renal insufficiency may be indolent or rapidly progressive and is usually closely associated with excretion of light chains. Therapy for the renal damage consists of adequate hydration, treatment of hypercalcemia and other metabolic abnormalities, and methods to decrease the production and renal excretion of abnormal paraproteins (for example, chemotherapy and/or plasmapheresis in patients with acute renal failure).

Patients with sickle cell disease may develop impaired urinary concentrating ability associated with polyuria, nocturia, and episodes of microscopic and gross hematuria. Gross hematuria requires investigation to rule out associated urinary tract disorders, followed by symptomatic treatment with hydration and transfusions to correct blood loss and increase the concentration of hemoglobin AA. Some patients develop a form of focal segmental glomerulosclerosis and the nephrotic syndrome. In patients with sickle cell disease, deformed erythrocytes obstruct the renal microcirculation. This leads to local ischemia and infarction, especially in a hypertonic, hypoxemic renal medulla. Areas of necrosis and interstitial fibrosis with eventual papillary necrosis also develop.

Although renal involvement is often asymptomatic in patients with sarcoidosis, patients may have mild proteinuria, sterile pyuria, and urine concentrating and acidifying defects. Rare patients present with acute renal failure and severe interstitial inflammation that may respond dramatically to glucocorticoid therapy. Renal biopsy specimens may show diffuse interstitial inflammatory infiltrates with giant cells and noncaseating granulomas or nephrocalcinosis secondary to hypercalcemia and hypercalciuria.

Genetic Disorders and Renal Disease

Genetic disorders may cause kidney disease either directly as a result of genetically mediated renal functional or morphologic abnormalities or indirectly as a result of genetically induced systemic disturbances in which the kidney is involved secondarily (Sessa) (Table 12).

Sessa A, ed. Hereditary Kidney Diseases. New York: S. Karger Publishing; 1997:1-217. UI: 9712796

TABLE 12 Kidney Diseases Caused by Genetic Disorders

Disease	Inheritance Mode	Gene Locus	Population Frequency
Polycystic kidney disease	Autosomal dominant (common) Autosomal recessive (rare)	Chromosomes 16 and 4	1:1000 1:40,000
Familial focal segmental glomerulosclerosis	Autosomal dominant (?)	Chromosome 19	–
Alport's syndrome	X-linked (80%)	Xq22	1:5000–10,000
	Autosomal recessive (10%)	2q35–37	1:5000–10,000
Benign familial hematuria (thin-basement membrane disease)	Autosomal dominant (carrier)	2q and 13q	–
Nephrogenic diabetes insipidus	Autosomal recessive		–
Bartter's syndrome	Autosomal recessive	Not known	1:2 million
Gitelman's syndrome	Autosomal recessive	Chromosome 16	?
Cystinuria	Autosomal recessive	Chromosome 2p	1:7000
Fabry's disease	X-linked	X q21, 22	1:40,000
Hyperoxaluria, types I, II, III	Autosomal recessive	2q36–37	–

p = short arm of chromosome; q = long arm of chromosome

Genetic Disorders Causing Direct Renal Effects

Polycystic Kidney Disease

Polycystic kidneys are characterized by countless epithelial-lined renal cysts scattered throughout the cortex and medulla of both kidneys. There are two major forms: Autosomal *dominant* polycystic kidney disease (ADPKD) and autosomal *recessive* polycystic kidney disease (ARPKD). ADPKD is usually diagnosed in patients who are 30 to 50 years old, whereas ARPKD is usually expressed at birth and is lethal during the neonatal period. ARPKD is caused by a mutation on chromosome 6 and is quite rare (1:40,000 live births).

KEY POINTS

- **Diagnostic clues to autosomal dominant polycystic kidney disease (ADPKD):**
  - **Age < 30 years: two renal cysts (unilateral/bilateral)**
  - **Age > 30 years: at least two cysts in each kidney**
  - **Family history of ADPKD**

ADPKD is a common cause of renal failure. In 95% of patients, it is caused by an abnormal gene on the short arm of chromosome 16. Most of the remaining patients have an abnormal gene on chromosome 4. Recent evidence suggests that a third gene may be implicated in this disease in a few patients. ADPKD occurs with a frequency of about 1:1000. It affects all races and ethnic groups. Early clinical manifestations include back and flank pain, hematuria, renal stones, hypertension, and urinary tract infections, all of which occur with increased frequency in patients with ADPKD. Approximately 50% of patients develop renal insufficiency before age 70 years, and renal function declines linearly over several years. ADPKD is associated with cerebral aneurysms (especially if there is a family history of aneurysm), with hepatic cysts in 40% to 60% of patients, with mitral and aortic valve prolapse, and with diverticular disease of the colon (Fick and Gabow).

Fick GM, Gabow PA. Hereditary and acquired cystic disease of the kidney. Kidney Int. 1994;46:951-64. UI: 95165749

Conlon PJ, Lynn K, Winn MP, Quarles LD, Bembe ML, Pericak-Vance M, et al. Spectrum of disease in familial focal and segmental glomerulosclerosis. Kidney Int. 1999;56:1863-71. UI: 20040884

Familial Focal Segmental Glomerulosclerosis

Several investigators have described the familial occurrence of focal segmental glomerulosclerosis. Both autosomal dominant and autosomal recessive inheritance have been reported. In the United States, 10% of families with several affected generations are black Americans, and 50% of families with affected individuals within a single generation are black Americans. Approximately 50% of patients progress to end-stage renal disease by 30 years of age (Conlon et al.).

Nephronophthisis–Medullary Cystic Disease Complex

These two related conditions are characterized by multiple cysts located in the corticomedullary junction and in the medulla. The cysts arise from the distal and collecting tubules. The disease causes tubular atrophy, interstitial inflammation and scarring, and eventually renal failure. Familial nephronophthisis is an autosomal recessive disorder that causes renal failure before the age of 20 years. Medullary cystic disease is an autosomal dominant disorder that causes renal failure in early adulthood. The initial clinical presentation of both disorders is marked by polyuria, polydipsia, nocturia (as a result of a renal concentrating disorder), and renal salt wasting, all of which are due to the tubular injury caused by the cystic and scarring process. Azotemia and end-stage renal disease follow.

Medullary Sponge Kidney

Medullary sponge kidney, which does not cause renal failure, is associated with hematuria, hypercalciuria (50% of patients), nephrocalcinosis, calcium stone disease, and hemihypertrophy. Familial occurrence accounts for many, although not most, cases. The diagnosis is made by an intravenous pyelogram showing small cystic outpouchings of the renal papillary ducts.

Alport's Syndrome

Alport's syndrome is an X-linked disorder in 80% of patients and an autosomal recessive disorder in approximately 10% of patients. Affected males develop hematuria, proteinuria, and renal failure in the second or third decade. The abnormal gene is on the long arm of chromosome 22 in the X-linked disorder and on the long arm of chromosome 2 in the autosomal recessive disorder. The gene defect causes a disorder of types IV and V collagen production and results in abnormalities of the ocular lens and glomerular basement membrane and hearing abnormalities (deafness). Affected heterozygous females have hematuria, but renal failure is uncommon.

Benign Familial Hematuria

Benign familial hematuria is a disorder of collagen synthesis that causes microscopic or gross hematuria and abnormally thin glomerular basement membranes. Genetic studies have suggested that this disorder represents a carrier state of the autosomal recessive form of Alport's syndrome. In contrast to Alport's syndrome, benign familial hematuria usually does not result in renal failure.

KEY POINTS

- Diagnostic clues to benign familial hematuria:
  - Onset during childhood
  - Unexplained microscopic or gross hematuria
  - Erythrocyte casts
  - Family history of hematuria
- Diagnostic clues to nephrogenic diabetes insipidus:
  - Onset during infancy or early childhood
  - Polyuria and thirst
  - Hypernatremia
- Diagnostic clues to Bartter's syndrome:
  - Onset during childhood or adolescence
  - Growth retardation
  - Hypokalemia
  - Normotension

Nephrogenic Diabetes Insipidus, Bartter's Syndrome, and Gitelman's Syndrome

Nephrogenic diabetes insipidus, Bartter's syndrome, and Gitelman's syndrome are genetically mediated disorders of renal tubular function. In patients with nephrogenic diabetes insipidus, tubular unresponsiveness to antidiuretic hormone causes urinary concentrating defects and polyuria. Abnormal chloride transporters in the ascending loop of Henle (in patients with Bartter's syndrome) and the distal tubule (in patients with Gitelman's syndrome) result in hypokalemia, hypochloremic metabolic alkalosis, and renal potassium wasting; however, blood pressure is usually normal.

Cystinuria

See later section on Nephrolithiasis.

Genetic Disorders Causing Systemic Abnormalities that Affect the Kidneys

Fabry's Disease

Fabry's disease is due to a deficiency of the enzyme α-galactosidase A that is caused by an abnormal gene on the long arm of the X chromosome (q21 and q22). Males are affected more often than females. The enzyme deficiency causes an accumulation of neutral glycophospholipid in endothelial, epithelial, and smooth muscle cells throughout the body. There is marked accumulation of glycophospholipid in the glomerular and tubular cells. Clinical features include proteinuria and renal failure, angiokeratomas of the skin, painful paresthesias of the hands, and premature coronary disease. Electron microscopy of the kidneys shows the characteristic inclusion bodies in the cytoplasm with concentric lamellation and a "zebra" or "onionskin" appearance. The same structures can be found by electron microscopic examination of spun urine sediment.

Primary Hyperoxaluria

Primary hyperoxaluria results from an inborn error of metabolism in which glyoxylate cannot be converted to glycine because of a deficiency of either glyoxylate aminotransferase or glyoxylate reductase in the liver. There are three genetic forms. Types I and II have similar clinical presentations. The type I disorder is most frequent and is caused by an abnormal gene on chromosome 2q36-37. The type III disorder is caused by excessive intestinal reabsorption of oxalate in the absence of any other gastrointestinal disease.

KEY POINTS

- Diagnostic clues to Fabry's disease:
  - Acroparesthesias
  - Cutaneous angiokeratomas
  - Proteinuria and azotemia
- Diagnostic clues to primary hyperoxaluria:
  - Calcium oxalate nephrolithiasis in childhood

Genetic Factors in Patients with Diabetic Nephropathy

Four lines of evidence support a genetic susceptibility for diabetic nephropathy: 1) the familial clustering of diabetic nephropathy in Pima Indians in whom the incidence of proteinuria in diabetic offspring is 14% if neither parent has proteinuria, 23% if one parent has diabetes mellitus and proteinuria, and 46% if both parents have diabetes mellitus and proteinuria; 2) the high association between a family history of hypertension and the development of diabetic nephropathy; 3) the similarity of renal lesions in siblings with diabetes mellitus; and 4) the influence of *ACE* gene and collagen gene polymorphisms.

Electrolytes

Case 9

A 22-year-old man with a 5-year history of type 1 diabetes mellitus develops a dental abscess. Two days after antibiotic therapy is started, he develops polyuria, nausea, vomiting, and dyspnea. Blood urea nitrogen is 56 mg/dL, and serum creatinine is 1.8 mg/dL. Serum sodium is 125 meq/L, potassium 3.6 meq/L, chloride 80 meq/L, and bicarbonate 10 meq/L. Plasma glucose is 975 mg/dL. Arterial blood gas studies (with the patient breathing room air) are pH 7.38, P_{CO_2} 17 mm Hg, and P_{O_2} 110 mm Hg.

Gennari FJ. Current concepts. Serum osmolality. Uses and limitations. N Engl J Med. 1984;310:102-5. UI: 84093415

Water Spaces, Osmolality, and Sodium

- What measured plasma osmolality would you expect for the patient in Case 9?
- What component of this patient's hyponatremia can be attributed to the hyperglycemia?
- If insulin is used to correct this patient's glucose concentration, will his extracellular fluid (ECF) volume increase, decrease, or stay the same? What serum sodium concentration would you expect after correction?
- What acid-base disorder(s) does this patient have?

Total Body Water = 60% Body Weight (BW)

ECF	ICF
20% (BW)	40% (BW)
Osmolality = 290 mosm/kg	Osmolality = 290 mosm/kg
Na = 145 meq/L	K = 145 meq/L

FIGURE 2
Normal distribution of water and electrolyte solutes.
In a 70-kg (154-lb) man, total body water is approximately 42 L, extracellular fluid (ECF) is 14 L, and intracellular fluid (ICF) is 28 L. The ECF includes plasma (about 3.5 L) and interstitial and transcellular water. The major solutes of ECF are sodium salts that are largely restricted to this compartment. Under normal circumstances, the ECF, plasma, or serum osmolality can be calculated as:

$$P_{osm} = 2 \times [Na]$$

The intracellular solutes are primarily potassium salts. Most cell membranes have very high water permeability so that water quickly moves across them rapidly to eliminate any osmotic gradient. Therefore, assume that the ECF and ICF osmolalities are equal. When the ECF or ICF osmolality is altered, water, and sometimes solute, shifts quickly reestablish the osmolal equality in these fluid spaces.

The normal distribution of water and electrolyte solutes and their contribution to ECF (and to plasma) osmolality are shown in Figure 2 (Gennari). Normally, sodium salts account for almost the entire ECF osmolality. When nonsodium solutes accumulate in the ECF, they contribute to osmolality in proportion to their molar concentrations. For example, high glucose and/or urea concentrations have the following effect:

$$P_{osm} = 2 \times [Na] + \frac{[BUN, mg/dL]}{2.8} + \frac{[Glucose, mg/dL]}{18} \quad \text{Equation 1}$$

where P_{osm} = plasma osmolality and BUN = blood urea nitrogen. (The constants 2.8 and 18 convert the [BUN] and [glucose] from mg/dL to mmol/L).

High glucose and urea levels have very different effects on water distribution and the plasma [Na]. High glucose levels are largely restricted to the ECF.

The attendant increase in ECF osmolality rapidly shifts water from the intracellular fluid (ICF) to the ECF. This simultaneously dilutes ECF and increases ICF solute concentrations and osmolality (Oster and Singer). The water shift continues until the ECF and the ICF osmolalities are equal. Each 100 mg/dL increase in [glucose] will reduce the [Na] by about 1.6 meq/L. Conversely, when hyperglycemia is corrected, water shifts from the ECF into the ICF, so that a 100 mg/dL reduction in [glucose] increases [Na] by about 1.6 meq/L. (Recent studies suggest that the correction factor may be somewhat higher.)

Oster JR, Singer I. Hyponatremia, hyposmolality, and hypotonicity: tables and fables. Arch Intern Med. 1999;159:333-6. UI: 99153376

The initial plasma osmolality of the patient in Case 9 should be about 324 mosm/kg H_2O. His [Na] should increase by about 14 meq/L, to 139 meq/L, after glucose correction, and his ECF will contract by 1 to 2 L. His acid-base abnormality is anion gap metabolic acidosis (ketoacidosis), metabolic alkalosis (probably due to vomiting), and respiratory alkalosis. This is explained in the following section on Acid-Base Disorders.

Mannitol, which is an osmotic diuretic used to treat cerebral edema, has similar size and compartmental distribution characteristics as glucose (in the absence of insulin) and has similar effects on salt and water distribution. In contrast, urea (a smaller molecule), rapidly penetrates most cell membranes. When urea levels increase, the concentrations of urea in the ICF and ECF are similar. Therefore, compartmental water shifts do not occur (this may not be true when ECF urea concentrations change rapidly). Other smaller neutral solutes such as ethanol, methanol, and ethylene glycol also readily penetrate cell membranes and, like urea, do not cause any water shift. The permeability properties of glycine are intermediate between glucose and urea. Glycine-containing solutions are used during transurethral prostatectomy, endometrial ablation, and arthroscopic procedures. Occasionally, large quantities of glycine irrigant are accidentally infused intravenously, or are absorbed, and may produce hyponatremia. This occurs for two reasons. First, glycine irrigation solutions are usually hypo-osmolal (approximately 200 mosm/kg H_2O). Second, to the extent that glycine is restricted to the ECF, it will cause water to shift from the ICF in a manner similar to mannitol or glucose.

Osmolal Gap

Case 10

A 56-year-old woman with a history of depression argues with her boyfriend and then attempts suicide by drinking a large glass of unknown "poison" that she found in the garage. Two hours later, she is brought to the emergency department. Blood urea nitrogen is 18 mg/dL. Serum sodium is 138 meq/L, potassium 5.0 meq/L, chloride 98 meq/L, and bicarbonate 15 meq/L. Plasma glucose is 110 mg/dL, and plasma osmolality is 330 mosm/kg H_2O. Urinalysis is normal.

Some molecules that can accumulate in the ECF and raise plasma osmolality are not sodium salts, glucose, or urea. Therefore, they are not included in equation 1. When such molecules accumulate in the ECF, the measured osmolality will exceed the osmolality calculated with equation 1. This difference is the "osmolal gap." Mannitol, glycine, ethanol, methanol, and ethylene glycol are all solutes that can produce an osmolal gap. The patient in Case 10 has an osmolal gap of 330 – 288 = 42. This suggests that ethanol, methanol, or ethylene glycol is the ingested poison. The serum bicarbonate of 15 meq/L and anion gap of 25 meq/L are more consistent with methanol or ethylene glycol ingestion. The absence of urine crystals is more consistent with methanol ingestion. (See following section on Acid-Base Disorders.)

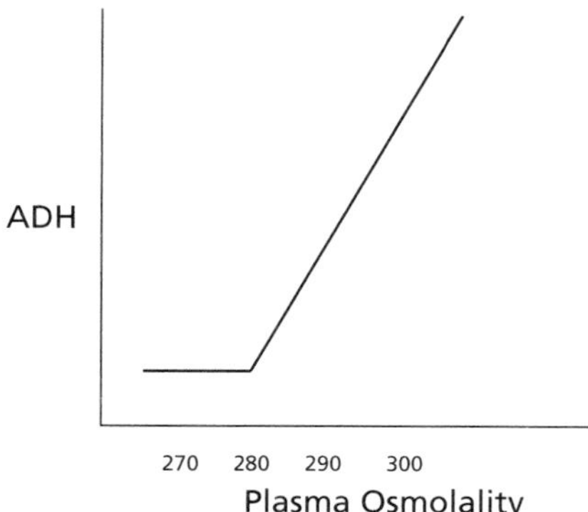

FIGURE 3
Plasma osmolality (mosm/kg H_2O) and release of antidiuretic hormone (ADH).

Adrogue HJ, Madias NE. Hyponatremia. N Engl J Med. 2000;342:1581-9. UI: 20267493

The coordinated actions of antidiuretic hormone (ADH), the renal concentrating–diluting system, and the ingestion of water maintain normal plasma osmolality and [Na]. When osmolality increases above 290 mosm/kg H_2O, ADH is released and thirst is triggered (Figure 3). ADH causes water reabsorption in the distal nephron and can increase urine osmolality to the range of 800 to 1200 mosm/kg H_2O. When plasma osmolality falls below 280 mosm/kg H_2O, secretion of ADH should stop. In the absence of ADH, maximally dilute urine (50–80 mosm/kg) is normally excreted. ADH can also be released independently of plasma osmolality in response to hypotension, a 7% to 10% decrease in plasma volume, vomiting, or a low effective arterial volume, which often complicates hepatic cirrhosis or congestive heart failure. A number of other nonosmotic factors, including dry mucous membranes, certain psychotropic medications, and high angiotensin levels, can also increase thirst.

Hyponatremia

Hyponatremia may be associated with normal, low, or high plasma osmolality (Adrogue and Madias). Hyponatremia with normal or increased osmolality can be caused by hyperglycemia or high mannitol concentrations (see above). The water that moves from the ICF into the ECF expands this space and reduces the sodium concentration. Hypo-osmolal hyponatremia indicates an excess of total body water relative to total body solute. The low ECF osmolality means that ICF osmolality is equally reduced. Cerebral edema may develop if water shifts into the brain ICF. Most patients with hypo-osmolal hyponatremia have high ADH levels and excrete inappropriately concentrated urine. Table 13 categorizes hypo-osmolal hyponatremia on the basis of ECF volume and effective intravascular volume status. The history, physical examination (with special attention to blood pressure, pulse, the presence of orthostatic changes, edema, ascites, crackles, etc.), measure of urinary [Na] and [osmolality], and determination of blood urea nitrogen and uric acid concentrations indicate the appropriate category and help to direct further evaluation and therapy. Although ADH levels can be measured, the measurement rarely narrows the differential diagnosis because the ADH concentration is usually increased.

In the volume-depleted patient with hyponatremia, administration of normal saline increases the glomerular filtration rate (GFR), increases the delivery of sodium and fluid to the distal tubules, and simultaneously inhibits ADH

TABLE 13 Evaluation of Hypo-osmolal Hyponatremia

	Total ECF Volume Status		
	Volume Depleted	**Euvolemic**	**Volume Expanded***
Clinical findings	Gastrointestinal fluid losses	SIADH	Congestive heart failure
	Third spacing	Hypothyroidism	Cirrhosis
	Adrenal insufficiency	Glucocorticoid deficiency	Nephrotic syndrome
	Renal salt-wasting		
Biochemical findings†			
Urinary sodium	< 10 meq/L‡	> 10 meq/L	< 10 meq/L
Urine osmolality	High	High	High
Plasma antidiuretic hormone	Elevated	Elevated	Elevated
Blood urea nitrogen	Elevated	< 10 mg/dL	Elevated
Serum uric acid	Elevated	< 4 mg/dL	Elevated

ECF = extracellular fluid, SIADH = syndrome of inappropriate antidiuretic hormone secretion
*Volume expanded in this context is defined as edema, ascites, and/or pulmonary congestion but low effective arterial blood volume.
†Assume no diuretic effect.
‡However, will be high with renal salt wasting.

release. This produces a water diuresis that corrects the hyponatremia. Patients with an expanded total ECF but a low effective arterial blood volume (for example, patients with congestive heart failure or cirrhosis) require therapy directed at the underlying organ dysfunction. Salt intake must usually be restricted in this group of patients. Water restriction is required when the [Na] is less than 125 meq/L. Loop diuretics can be used to promote natriuresis and to simultaneously reduce the maximal renal concentrating capacity.

Most patients with euvolemic hyponatremia have the syndrome of inappropriate antidiuretic hormone secretion (SIADH). The major causes of SIADH are pulmonary diseases, central nervous system dysfunction, drugs, and carcinomas, especially small cell lung cancer. Hypothyroidism and cortisol deficiency also produce euvolemic hyponatremia and must be ruled out before a diagnosis of SIADH is established.

The treatment of hyponatremia is directed by its severity, cause, chronicity, and associated symptoms. If the causative pathologic findings cannot be eliminated, the low sodium level itself may require therapy. Chronic moderately symptomatic hyponatremia (which usually develops in outpatients) is treated conservatively with the goal of correcting the [Na] over many days (Kumar and Berl). Water restriction is the cornerstone of therapy for patients with chronic moderate hyponatremia. Adjunctive therapy includes the administration of loop diuretics, which reduce maximal renal concentrating capacity, combined with liberal intake of sodium chloride. This strategy may reduce the requirement for severe water restriction. Demeclocycline can be used to produce reversible nephrogenic diabetes insipidus, thereby promoting renal free water excretion. Administration of oral nonpeptide ADH antagonists (aquaretics) to treat various chronic hyponatremic conditions is currently being studied. Overly aggressive and too rapid correction of chronic hyponatremia can result in a catastrophic neurologic complication called central pontine and extrapontine myelinolysis. This often fatal disorder is very unlikely if the rate of sodium correction is less than 0.5 meq/h and the absolute level of acute sodium correction is kept below 120 meq/L.

Kumar S, Berl T. Sodium. Lancet. 1998;352:220-8. UI: 98346757

Acute symptomatic hyponatremia occurs more commonly in hospitalized patients. When the [Na] falls rapidly to less than 120 meq/L, nausea, vomiting, irritability, mental confusion, and seizures may occur, and an acute [Na] reduction below 110 meq/L may result in coma and death. Women of childbearing age may be especially susceptible to a unique form of severe, and often fatal, acute postoperative hyponatremia. The symptomatic acute hyponatremia syndromes require prompt and aggressive therapy. Hypertonic (3% = 517 meq/L) saline may be infused to increase the [Na]. The quantity of NaCl required to increase the plasma [Na] is calculated by the following equation:

$$\text{meq Na required} = \text{total body water} \times \Delta[\text{Na}]$$
$$\text{meq Na required} = 0.6 \times \text{weight}_{kg} \times \Delta[\text{Na}] \qquad \text{Equation 2}$$

Although infused sodium is largely restricted to the ECF, total body water (TBW) is used in this calculation because any change in ECF [Na] produces a rapid water shift from the ICF. This calculation does not consider ongoing urinary, gastrointestinal, or insensible free water or electrolyte loss. Thus, plasma electrolytes must be monitored frequently during such treatment, especially if the urine output is large. Loop diuretics may also be used to increase free water excretion and to prevent ECF volume overload. A reasonable therapeutic goal for the partial correction of acute, severe, symptomatic hyponatremia is a [Na] increase of about 15 to 20 meq/L during the first 24 hours of therapy.

A disorder termed pseudohyponatremia is diagnosed primarily when laboratories use flame photometers to measure sodium and is caused by lipid displacement artifacts. However, this disorder is seldom encountered today because of the use of ion-specific electrodes.

Hypernatremia

Adrogue HJ, Madias NE. Hypernatremia. N Engl J Med. 2000;342:1493-9. UI: 20256709

A plasma [Na] greater than 145 meq/L defines hypernatremia (and hyperosmolality) (Adrogue and Madias). Hypernatremia usually develops when large volumes of fluids containing relatively low electrolyte concentrations (Na + K < 140 meq/L) are lost from the body. The losses may be renal, gastrointestinal, and insensible. Less commonly, hypernatremia is due to the infusion of hypertonic NaCl or $NaHCO_3$. Hypothalamic sensors detect the hypernatremia and normally trigger thirst and the synthesis and release of ADH. If ADH secretion and/or the renal response to ADH is abnormal, thirst and access to water will still usually prevent the development of severe hypernatremia. Therefore, persistent hypernatremia also indicates an abnormal thirst mechanism or an inability to ingest sufficient water. Hypernatremia produces lethargy, weakness, and irritability and can progress to seizures, coma, and death. The symptoms reflect the severity and rapidity of the development of the hypernatremia. The causes of hypernatremia are listed in Table 14.

When hypernatremia exists, the urine osmolality should be high. A low urine osmolality indicates malfunction of the ADH/renal concentrating mechanisms. Causes include defective ADH synthesis and/or release (central diabetes insipidus), accelerated peripheral ADH destruction (a rare disorder that occurs in some pregnant patients), or a defective renal response to ADH (nephrogenic diabetes insipidus). Some forms of central and nephrogenic dia-

TABLE 14 Causes of Hypernatremia
Increased Water Loss
Insensible
Burns
Fever/heat
Mechanical ventilation/hyperventilation
Gastrointestinal loss
Vomiting/nasogastric tube suction
Diarrhea
Renal loss
Central diabetes insipidus
Nephrogenic diabetes insipidus
Osmotic diuresis
Reduced Water Intake
Hypothalamic dysfunction
Reduced thirst
Essential hypernatremia?
Inability to drink water
Comatose patient
Infant not given adequate water
Hypertonic Infusions
Saline/sodium bicarbonate
Water Shift Out of Extracellular Fluid Compartment
Seizure/extreme exercise (water shifts into muscle cells)
Gastrointestinal bleeding with intraluminal protein catabolism (water shifts into lumen of intestine)

betes insipidus are inherited. More commonly, these disorders are acquired conditions. Acquired central diabetes insipidus may be due to infiltrative or granulomatous diseases (such as sarcoidosis), trauma, neoplasm, neurosurgery, or severe hypoxia. Patients with central diabetes insipidus will rapidly concentrate their urine in response to administration of ADH or the synthetic analog desmopressin (DDAVP). Such a response represents both a positive diagnostic test and appropriate therapy and differentiates these patients from those with nephrogenic diabetes insipidus in whom vasopressin administration produces no increase in urine concentration.

Acquired nephrogenic diabetes insipidus can be caused by several drugs (lithium, demeclocycline), chronic hypokalemia, hypercalcemia, sickle cell trait and disease, and amyloidosis. Loop diuretics also produce a renal concentrating defect. In contrast to patients with central diabetes insipidus, those with nephrogenic diabetes insipidus will not respond to ADH or DDAVP. Osmotic diuresis can also cause increased renal water loss with an inadequate renal concentrating response. Hospitalized patients may develop hypernatremia as a result of a urea osmotic diuresis caused by high protein intake, gastrointestinal bleeding (absorption of digested blood proteins), and/or glucocorticoid therapy (accelerated catabolism). Again, it should be stressed that hypernatremia should not occur if the patient is awake, can sense thirst, and has access to water.

Hypernatremia usually represents an absolute water deficit. Therefore, therapy requires water replacement and, when possible, correction or treatment of the underlying disorder. The water deficit can be calculated by the following formula:

$$\text{Water deficit} = (0.6)\,(\text{total body weight}_{kg})\left(\frac{[\text{Na}]}{140} - 1\right) \qquad \text{Equation 3}$$

Again, note that total body water is used in this calculation for the same reasons discussed in relation to equation 2. Whenever possible, water deficits should be replaced via the oral or gastric route. If intravenous replacement is required, 5% dextrose in water or $\frac{1}{4}$ NaCl can be used. The plasma glucose concentration must be carefully monitored when dextrose-containing fluids are administered because hyperglycemia may occur. This can cause a glucose osmotic diuresis that results in "chasing one's tail," as urine output progressively increases and the intravenous 5% dextrose in water infusion rate is increased to match output. About 50% of the water deficit should be replaced in the first 24 hours of therapy. Overly rapid water replacement can cause cerebral edema.

Always evaluate and address the intravascular volume status of the patient with hypernatremia. Patients with intravascular volume depletion (for example, those with hypotension or orthostasis) may require immediate ECF expansion, and isotonic NaCl may be the ideal initial fluid for these patients. The water deficit can be addressed after restoration of ECF volume. Conversely, some patients with hypernatremia will be volume expanded, for example, after hypertonic salts have been infused, and may require diuretic therapy as well as water replacement.

KEY POINTS

- High glucose or mannitol levels produce hyponatremia as a result of a shift of water out of cells that expands the extracellular fluid (ECF) volume. High blood urea nitrogen (BUN) concentrations increase osmolality but usually do not cause water shifts or sodium concentration changes. Methanol, ethylene glycol, and/or ethanol increase the measured osmolality and also do not cause any water shift.
- Hyponatremia is usually associated with an inappropriately high urine osmolality and elevated antidiuretic hormone (ADH) levels. This may be due to the syndrome of inappropriate antidiuretic hormone secretion (SIADH), volume depletion, or an edema-forming condition such as congestive heart failure, cirrhosis, or nephrotic syndrome.
- Before making a diagnosis of SIADH, rule out ECF volume depletion, hypothyroidism, and glucocorticoid deficiency.
- Acute symptomatic hyponatremia should be rapidly corrected to a sodium concentration of about 125 meq/L, but chronic hyponatremia should be corrected slowly (< 0.5 meq/h).
- Always address ECF volume deficits first regardless of the plasma osmolality.

Potassium Metabolism

Potassium is the principal cation of the ICF, where its concentration is approximately 150 meq/L. The concentration of K in the ECF and plasma is much lower, between 3.5 and 5.0 meq/L. Sodium/potassium adenosine triphosphatase (Na/K-ATPase) pumps in cell membranes and the ionic permeability characteristics of the cell membranes maintain this very large transcellular gradient. This transmembrane [K] gradient is the principal determinant of the transcellular resting potential gradient (about –90 mV; the cell interior is negative). Normal cellular function requires maintenance of the ECF [K] within a relatively narrow range.

Adults ingest 50 to 100 meq of potassium daily and under normal circumstances excrete an equal quantity in the urine. Renal potassium excretion is primarily determined by secretion in the distal renal tubules. Potassium secretion at that site is affected by the volume of fluid and the quantity of sodium traversing the distal tubules, the permeability characteristics of the anions accompanying the sodium (chloride versus bicarbonate versus organic anions), aldosterone activity and responsiveness, acid-base status, the serum [K], and intracellular [K] stores. The relationship between ingested (and infused) potassium and excreted potassium represents the external potassium balance. Internal potassium balance, which is responsible for the minute to minute regulation of the ECF [K], is a function of the transcellular gradient. Insulin, β_2-agonists, and bicarbonate drive potassium into cells. High ECF tonicity (mainly hyperglycemia), acidemia (mainly hyperchloremic acidosis), and leaky cell membranes (rhabdomyolysis, hemolysis, Na/K-ATPase inhibition) cause potassium to shift from cells into the ECF (Sterns et al.; Halperin and Kamel).

Sterns RH, Cox M, Feig PU, Singer I. Internal potassium balance and the control of the plasma potassium concentration. Medicine (Baltimore). 1981;60:339-54. UI: 82012835

Halperin ML, Kamel KS. Potassium. Lancet. 1998;352:135-40. UI: 98336038

Hypokalemia

Very low potassium intake, excessive potassium loss, and/or a potassium shift from the ECF into the ICF may cause hypokalemia. Increased urinary potassium excretion indicates that primary or secondary renal potassium wasting contributes to the hypokalemia, whereas urinary potassium conservation indicates extrarenal potassium loss or an internal potassium shift. Measurement of 24-hour urinary potassium excretion or a spot urinary potassium concentration can be a useful discriminator (Table 15). Although low dietary potassium intake is often a contributing factor, it is rarely the sole cause of hypokalemia.

Hypokalemia can produce muscle cramps, ileus, rhabdomyolysis, and respiratory paralysis. Electrocardiographic abnormalities include flat or inverted T waves, U waves, and both supraventricular and ventricular arrhythmias, especially in patients receiving digoxin. Hypokalemia blunts insulin secretion and can produce hyperglycemia. Chronic hypokalemia is a cause of nephrogenic diabetes insipidus and may also cause multiple small renal cysts.

Supplemental potassium salts are indicated when external potassium losses cause hypokalemia (Cohn et al.). When possible, oral potassium salts should be used. KCl is the appropriate salt to administer when hypokalemia is associated with metabolic alkalosis. Salts such as potassium citrate are alkalinizing and are best used to treat hypokalemia associated with metabolic acidosis (for example,

Cohn JN, Kowey PR, Whelton PK, Prisant LM. New guidelines for potassium replacement in clinical practice: a contemporary review by the National Council on Potassium in Clinical Practice. Arch Intern Med. 2000;160:2429-36. UI: 20435208

TABLE 15 Differential Diagnosis of Hypokalemia

High Urinary [K] – Renal Loss*	Low Urinary [K]†
Metabolic acidosis	Gastrointestinal losses
Renal tubular acidosis	Diarrhea
Distal (untreated)	Laxative abuse
Proximal (treated)	Internal shifts
Drugs	Periodic paralysis
Acetazolamide	Insulin
Metabolic alkalosis	β_2-Agonists
(See following section on Acid–Base Disorders)	Alkalosis
	Dietary deficiency

*Greater than 20 meq/24 h or 20 meq/L.
†Less than 20 meq/24 h or 20 meq/L.

renal tubular acidosis or diarrhea). When potassium salts cannot be administered orally, they may be infused intravenously. Generally, the [K] of intravenous fluid should not exceed 40 meq/L, and the intravenous infusion rate of potassium should not exceed 20 to 40 meq/h. It is imperative to monitor serum [K] frequently during intravenous replacement because hyperkalemia can develop before potassium stores have been repleted. Total body deficits are difficult to predict. Generally, the deficit is about 200 to 400 meq when the serum [K] is 3.0 meq/L and about 400 to 800 meq when the serum [K] is 2.0 meq/L. Exogenous potassium supplements are not usually required when hypokalemia is due to an internal shift. However, if a shift has produced severe and symptomatic hypokalemia, some exogenous potassium may be used to ameliorate symptoms.

Always consider the possibility of coexisting hypomagnesemia when patients have severe hypokalemia. Potassium and magnesium are both intracellular anions and are often lost together. Magnesium replacement is important because magnesium depletion increases renal potassium excretion and thereby makes potassium replacement more difficult.

Hyperkalemia

The development of hyperkalemia is opposed by a shift of potassium from the ECF into cells and by increased renal potassium excretion. Hyperkalemia may occur as a result of abnormalities in one or both of these regulatory systems. However, chronic hyperkalemia is almost invariably associated with reduced renal potassium excretion.

Impaired renal potassium excretion may be caused by acute or chronic renal failure, diminished urine flow rates, impaired aldosterone production, reduced renal aldosterone responsiveness, and several other renal tubule potassium secretory defects. Table 16 lists the most common causes of impaired renal potassium excretion.

Increased potassium loads can be delivered to the ECF because of excessive dietary intake, intravenous infusions, and/or potassium shifts from the ICF to the ECF. Excessive dietary potassium will rarely cause hyperkalemia unless renal potassium excretion is simultaneously impaired. Potassium is shifted out of the ICF when cell membranes are disrupted (for example, rhabdomyolysis or hemolysis), when ECF osmolality is markedly increased (for example, hyperglycemia), when metabolic acidosis develops (especially hyperchloremic metabolic acidosis), and when insulin or β_2-adrenergic activity is impaired or blocked.

Severe hyperkalemia often causes cardiac toxicity. The electrocardiogram shows peaked T waves, flattened P waves, and a widened QRS complex that can progress to ventricular arrhythmias, a "sine wave," and ventricular fibrillation. Hyperkalemia reduces the transmembrane potassium gradient, which causes muscle weakness and may lead to flaccid paralysis.

Treatment options for patients with acute hyperkalemia include:

- Antagonizing the cardiac toxic effects with intravenous calcium salts.
- Shifting ECF potassium into cells by administering glucose, insulin, and/or β_2-adrenergic agonists. (The β_2-adrenergic agonist albuterol is available only in aerosolized form in the United States.) Sodium bicarbonate is also used to shift potassium into cells but is not very effective in patients with normal acid-base status.
- Increasing potassium excretion via the kidneys by expanding ECF volume and administering kaliuretic diuretics and via the gastrointestinal tract by inducing diarrhea and administering the potassium-binding resin, sodium polystyrene sulfonate. Hemodialysis or peritoneal dialysis is used to remove potassium when hyperkalemia develops in patients with renal failure.

TABLE 16 Causes of Hyperkalemia

Increased intake
Shift from intracellular to extracellular fluid compartment:
Ex-vivo – pseudohyperkalemia
Metabolic acidosis (especially hyperchloremic)
β-Adrenergic blockade
Insulin deficiency/resistance
Hyperosmolality/hyperglycemia
Rhabdomyolysis
Hyperkalemic periodic paralysis
Arginine hydrochloride infusion
Succinylcholine
Digoxin overdose
Reduced renal excretion
Renal insufficiency/failure
Hypoaldosteronism
Aldosterone resistance (inherited, acquired, drug related)
Type IV renal tubular acidosis

Treatment of chronic hyperkalemia includes dietary potassium restriction, avoidance of drugs that impair renal potassium excretion, and, when appropriate, the administration of kaliuretic diuretics or exogenous mineralocorticoids (Weiner and Wingo; Ponce et al.).

Spurious hyperkalemia (pseudohyperkalemia) occurs when serum [K] increases in the test tube as a result of ex-vivo hemolysis or when the leukocyte or platelet count is markedly elevated and potassium is released during blood coagulation. These forms of pseudohyperkalemia can often be avoided by measuring [K] in plasma rather than serum.

Weiner ID, Wingo CS. Hyperkalemia: a potential silent killer. J Am Soc Nephrol. 1998;9:1535-43. UI: 98361143

Ponce SP, Jennings AE, Madias NE, Harrington JT. Drug-induced hyperkalemia. Medicine (Baltimore). 1985; 64:357-70. UI: 86039762

KEY POINTS

- A urine K concentration will help differentiate renal or extrarenal K loss in patients with hypokalemia.
- Chronic hypokalemia often produces polyuria due to nephrogenic diabetes insipidus.
- When severe hyperkalemia produces cardiac toxicity, intravenous calcium salts should first be given, followed by maneuvers to shift K into cells and to remove K from the body.

Phosphorus and Magnesium Metabolism

Serum phosphorus and magnesium concentrations are tightly controlled. Balance is determined by the interplay between intake, gastrointestinal absorption and secretion, and urinary excretion. Circulating levels are affected by the distribution of these ions between the ICF and ECF compartments. Development of persistent hypophosphatemia or hypomagnesemia generally requires a combination of two of the following: diminished intake, a shift from the ECF into the ICF compartment, decreased gastrointestinal absorption, and/or increased urinary excretion (Weisinger and Bellorin-Font).

Weisinger JR, Bellorin-Font E. Magnesium and phosphorus. Lancet. 1998;352:391-6. UI: 98382044

Hypophosphatemia

The serum phosphorus concentration does not always reflect total body phosphorus stores because most inorganic phosphorus is intracellular. Hypophosphatemia may result from renal disorders (for example, Fanconi's syndrome, familial hypophosphatemic rickets, X-linked hypophosphatemic rickets, oncogenic hypophosphatemia, or hypophosphatemia after renal transplantation). Hypophosphatemia may also be caused by hormonal alterations (for example, hyperparathyroidism) or pharmacologic effects (for example, alcohol) that result in decreased tubular reabsorption and excessive urinary excretion of phosphorus. Acute hypophosphatemia may also result from movement of ECF phosphorus into the ICF compartment, as occurs in patients with extensive burns. Hypophosphatemia is worsened by decreased nutritional intake, gastrointestinal disease, or vitamin D deficiency. An elevated urinary phosphorus concentration differentiates abnormal renal tubular handling of phosphorus from nutritional causes and internal shifts.

Severe hypophosphatemia (serum phosphorus level < 1 mg/dL) may be associated with the phosphorus depletion syndrome, which causes hematologic abnormalities (hemolytic anemia, impaired leukocyte function, and platelet disorders), myopathy, and metabolic encephalopathy. The effects have been attributed to depletion of intracellular ATP stores. When chronically malnourished patients are fed without administering adequate phosphorus, intracellular phosphorus stores may decrease precipitously. The phosphorus depletion syndrome is encountered in patients with chronic alcoholism, those with poor nutritional intake, and those with alcoholic ketoacidosis. Phosphorus shifts into the ICF compartment as a result of respiratory alkalosis can exacerbate the disorder. Diabetes mellitus may be associated with phosphorus depletion because polyuria, glucosuria, ketonuria, and acidemia increase urinary phosphorus excretion.

Either whole or skim milk is an excellent source of oral phosphorus. Fleet enema preparations, which contain sodium phosphate, can also be given orally three to four times a day as a source of phosphorus. Sometimes phosphorus must be administered intravenously, especially to symptomatic patients with serum phosphorus levels less than 1 mg/dL. However, hypocalcemia, metastatic calcification, and acute renal failure are adverse effects of parenteral phosphorus. When patients are treated with intravenous phosphorus, concentrations of calcium, phosphorus, and creatinine should be closely monitored.

Hyperphosphatemia

Administration of phosphorus by oral, intravenous, or rectal routes can produce hyperphosphatemia. Hypoparathyroidism, pseudohypoparathyroidism, acromegaly or growth hormone administration, and tumor cell lysis or rhabdomyolysis can also result in hyperphosphatemia. When the GFR falls below 25% to 30% of normal, the ability to excrete phosphorus in the urine lags behind gastrointestinal absorption, and hyperphosphatemia generally develops.

Hypomagnesemia

Magnesium depletion may be due to decreased intake, accelerated gastrointestinal or renal losses, redistribution out of the ECF, or multiple combinations of these derangements. The malabsorption syndromes, steatorrhea, chronic vomiting, nasogastric tube suction, and diarrhea all accelerate gastrointestinal excretion of magnesium. Chronic thiazide and loop diuretic use, primary hyperaldosteronism and other syndromes of sustained volume expansion, hypophosphatemia, alcohol withdrawal, and certain renal toxins (including cisplatin, amphotericin B, cyclosporine, aminoglycoside antibiotics, and pentamidine) increase urine magnesium excretion. Several inherited renal tubular defects, such as Gitelman's syndrome, cause renal magnesium wasting and hypomagnesemia. Redistribution of magnesium out of the ECF occurs with oral or intravenous refeeding of chronically malnourished patients and during the treatment of patients with uncontrolled diabetes mellitus. Large quantities of magnesium are often deposited in the skeleton following parathyroidectomy ("hungry bone syndrome") and precipitate as magnesium soaps in patients with severe pancreatitis. Decreased magnesium intake will exacerbate all of these disorders (Quamme).

Quamme GA. Renal magnesium handling: new insights in understanding old problems. Kidney Int. 1997;52:1180-95. UI: 98011743

Magnesium depletion and hypomagnesemia occur commonly in patients with chronic alcoholism, in patients with serious gastrointestinal disorders, and in 60% to 65% of patients in intensive care units. Hypomagnesemia is very common following liver transplantation.

Hypocalcemia and hypokalemia frequently complicate magnesium depletion. These chemical abnormalities are refractory to replacement therapy until the magnesium levels are restored. Hypocalcemia results from the combination of skeletal resistance to parathyroid hormone action and the abnormal synthesis and release of parathyroid hormone from the parathyroid glands. Hypokalemia is primarily due to accelerated renal potassium excretion.

The clinical manifestations of hypomagnesemia include lethargy, anorexia, nausea, tetany, and convulsions. Magnesium depletion may also produce cardiac arrhythmias, especially in patients who are receiving digoxin. It is often not clear what component of these abnormalities is due to hypomagnesemia per se and what is secondary to the associated hypokalemia or hypocalcemia.

Serum magnesium concentrations may not accurately reflect total body magnesium stores. Magnesium retention studies (measurement of the fraction of an administered intravenous magnesium load that is excreted over a defined period) may be the best indicator of a depleted state. When renal function is normal and magnesium stores are adequate, an intravenous magnesium load is rapidly (within 24 hours) excreted into the urine. Magnesium depletion causes the retention of 25% to 50% of the administered load. However, renal insufficiency or a renal tubular magnesium wasting defect may invalidate interpretation of a magnesium retention study.

The typical magnesium deficit in a depleted adult is 75 to 150 meq. Since up to 50% of an administered magnesium load will still be excreted into the urine of depleted patients with normal renal function, a total replacement dose of 150 to 300 meq may be required.

Moderate magnesium deficiency may be treated with oral magnesium salts. However, magnesium is poorly absorbed by the gastrointestinal tract, and large doses of magnesium salts produce diarrhea. Therefore, severe deficits usually require parenteral replacement. A 2-ml ampule of $MgSO_4 \bullet 7H_2O$ 50% contains 1 g of $MgSO_4$ = 98 mg = 8 meq of elemental Mg. Based on the above discussion, a total dose of 8 to 12 g of $MgSO_4$ (64 to 96 meq of Mg or 8 to 12 2-mL ampules of 50% $MgSO_4$) may be required (unless renal function is impaired).

Hypermagnesemia

The normal kidney efficiently excretes magnesium; therefore, hypermagnesemia rarely develops in patients with normal renal function. However, a very large magnesium load can produce short-term magnesium toxicity in a patient with a normal GFR. Sources of exogenous magnesium include intravenous infusions (used to treat toxemia of pregnancy or to correct hypomagnesemia), oral salts (for example, Epsom salt, magnesium citrate, milk of magnesia), and magnesium salt enemas. High magnesium blood levels cause dose-dependent neuromuscular toxicity that begins with diminished deep tendon reflexes and progresses to flaccid paralysis and respiratory failure. Bradycardia, hypotension, and heart block are due to the calcium channel blocking effects of hypermagnesemia.

Most of the acute toxicity of hypermagnesemia is rapidly (within minutes) antagonized by an intravenous infusion of calcium. Restoration of normal [Mg] can be achieved with ECF expansion and loop diuretics if renal function is near normal. When severe hypermagnesemia develops in a patient with poor renal function, hemodialysis or peritoneal dialysis can efficiently and rapidly normalize the blood [Mg].

KEY POINTS

- Consider hypomagnesemia whenever severe hypocalcemia and/or hypokalemia is found.
- Magnesium depletion is common in patients with malabsorption, chronic diarrhea, and/or chronic alcohol abuse.
- The acute neuromuscular toxicity of hypermagnesemia is promptly reversed by intravenous infusion of calcium salts.

Acid-Base Disorders

The Henderson-Hasselbalch equation shows the relationship between the pH, arterial carbon dioxide pressure (P_{CO_2}), and bicarbonate (HCO_3).

$$pH = 6.1 + \log \frac{[HCO_3]}{(0.03)\ P_{CO_2}}$$

A primary rise in arterial P_{CO_2} (respiratory acidosis) or fall in plasma [HCO_3] (metabolic acidosis) reduces pH, whereas a primary fall in arterial P_{CO_2} (respiratory alkalosis) or rise in plasma [HCO_3] (metabolic alkalosis) increases pH. Each primary disorder should trigger a compensatory response that returns the pH toward normal. The magnitude of each compensatory response is predictable, as shown in Table 17 (Gluck; Adrogue and Madias, parts 1 and 2).

Gluck SL. Acid-base. Lancet. 1998; 352:474-9. UI: 98372501

Adrogue HJ, Madias NE. Management of life-threatening acid-base disorders. First of two parts. N Engl J Med. 1998;338:26-34. UI: 98069943

Adrogue HJ, Madias NE. Management of life-threatening acid-base disorders. Second of two parts. N Engl J Med. 1998;338:107-11 UI: 98069970

Metabolic Acidosis

Case 11

A 47-year-old man has a 3-day history of severe diarrhea and comes to the emergency department because of weakness, dyspnea, and dizziness. On physical examination, his supine blood

TABLE 17 Acid-Base Disorders and Compensatory Responses

Disorder	H^+	pH	HCO_3	Arterial Blood Pco_2	Adaptive Response	Time for Adaptation
Metabolic acidosis	↑	↓	↓↓	↓	$\Delta Pco_2 = (1.5) HCO_3 + 8$ $\Delta Pco_2 = HCO_3 + 15$	12 to 24 h
Metabolic alkalosis	↓	↑	↑↑	↑	$Pco_2 = > 40$ mm Hg, usually < 55	24 to 36 h
Respiratory acidosis						
Acute	↑	↓	↑	↑↑	$\Delta HCO_3 = 0.1 \Delta Pco_2$	Minutes to hours
Chronic	↑	↓	↑	↑↑	$\Delta HCO_3 = 0.3 \Delta Pco_2$	Days
Respiratory alkalosis						
Acute	↓	↑	↓	↓↓	$\Delta HCO_3 = 0.2 \Delta Pco_2$	Minutes to hours
Chronic	↓	↑	↓	↓↓	$\Delta HCO_3 = 0.4 \Delta Pco_2$	Days

Double arrows indicate the primary disturbance.

pressure is 100/70 mm Hg, and his supine pulse rate is 110/min. When the patient sits, his systolic blood pressure decreases to 80 mm Hg, and his pulse rate increases to 130/min. Blood urea nitrogen is 30 mg/dL, serum creatinine 1.7 mg/dL, sodium 130 meq/L, potassium 3.2 meq/L, chloride 100 meq/L, and bicarbonate 10 meq/L. Arterial blood gas studies (with the patient breathing room air) are pH 7.24, Pco_2 24 mm Hg, Po_2 105 mm Hg, and bicarbonate 9 meq/L.

Metabolic acidosis is a pathologic process that causes a primary decrease in plasma [HCO_3]. One or more of the following mechanisms are usually responsible: 1) accelerated loss of alkali into the stool or urine; 2) increased acid loads that exceed the normal acid excretory or metabolic capacity; and 3) decreased ability of the kidneys to excrete acid.

It is helpful to divide the metabolic acidoses into those with an increased anion gap (AG) and those with increased chloride concentration [Cl]. Figure 4 shows how the anion gap is calculated, and Figure 5 illustrates why the [AG], the [Cl], or both, must increase when metabolic acidosis develops. Note that the quantitative increase in [AG] and/or [Cl] should approximate the quantitative reduction in [HCO_3].

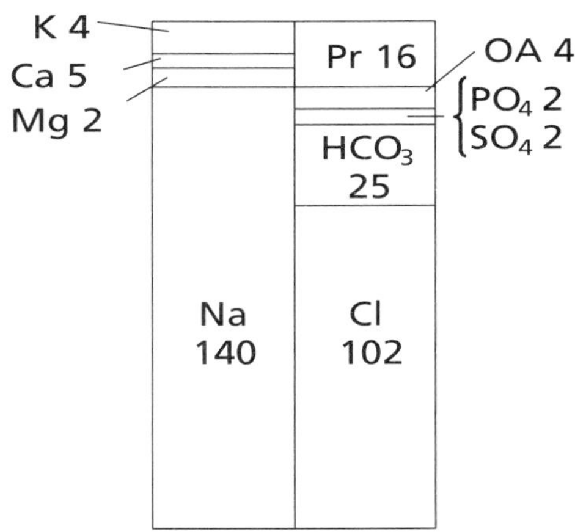

AG 8
HCO3 25
Na 140
Cl 102

$$AG = Na - (Cl + HCO_3)$$

FIGURE 4
Calculation of the anion gap (AG).
The sum of all the anions and all the cations in serium must be equal (all measured in meq/L). If only [Na], [Cl], and [HCO_3] are used, then an anion gap of 8 to12 will be found.
AG = anion gap; OA = organic anions;
Pr = proteins, mainly albumin

FIGURE 5
[AG] and [Cl] in metabolic acidosis.
When any relatively strong acid, such as HX, is added to the ECF, the H^+ dissociates and combines with HCO_3^- to form H_2CO_3 which then dehydrates to generate H_2O and CO_2. The X^- remains and can be considered NaX. If HX is HCl, then the increase in [Cl] will match the fall in HCO_3^-; if X^- is any non-HCl acid (such as lactic acid), the fall in HCO_3^- will be matched by a similar increase in the anion gap. External loss of $NaHCO_3$ also produces a hyperchloremic metabolic acidosis.
AG = anion gap, ECF = extracellular fluid

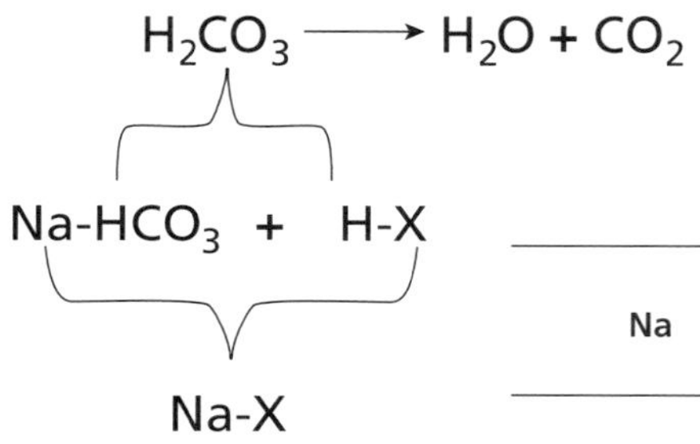

$$H_2CO_3 \longrightarrow H_2O + CO_2$$

$$Na\text{-}HCO_3 + H\text{-}X \rightarrow Na\text{-}X$$

	NORMAL	NORMAL AG METABOLIC ACIDOSIS (HYPERCHLOREMIC)	HIGH AG METABOLIC ACIDOSIS
Na	140	140	140
Cl	105	115	105
HCO_3	25	15	15
ANION GAP	10	10	20
LACTATE	1	1	11

The patient described in Case 11 has metabolic acidosis with appropriate respiratory compensation. The reduction in [HCO_3] is probably about 15 meq/L (having fallen from a normal level of 24 meq/L to 9 meq/L). His [AG] is 20 meq/L [130 – (100 + 10)]. In a patient with simple anion gap acidosis, the reduction in [HCO_3] is approximately equal to the increase in the anion gap (Emmett and Narins). For the patient in Case 11, if his baseline [AG] was 12 meq/L, then his [AG] has increased by about 8 meq/L. Thus the increase in [AG] accounts for only part of the [HCO_3] reduction. Therefore, he probably has both anion gap and hyperchloremic metabolic acidosis. His [Cl] of 100 meq/L is high relative to a [Na] of 130 meq/L. The hyponatremia is probably due to extracellular fluid (ECF) volume contraction combined with continued water intake. Hypokalemia results from loss of potassium in the stool (see Tables 13 and 15).

Emmett M, Narins RG. Clinical use of the anion gap. Medicine (Baltimore). 1977;56:38-54. UI: 77099376

Hyperchloremic Metabolic Acidosis

When metabolic acidosis reduces the [HCO_3] and the [AG] remains normal, the patient has hyperchloremic metabolic acidosis (chloride concentration relative to the sodium concentration is high). Hyperchloremic metabolic acidosis develops in one of two ways: 1) fluids containing high concentrations of sodium bicarbonate ($NaHCO_3$), or potential $NaHCO_3$ (see below) are lost from the ECF or 2) HCl , or potential HCl, is added to the ECF. Any organic sodium salt that can be metabolized to $NaHCO_3$ represents potential $NaHCO_3$. For example, sodium lactate, sodium citrate, sodium acetate, and sodium butyrate all generate $NaHCO_3$ when the organic anion is metabolized to nonionized substances such as glucose or CO_2 and H_2O. Chloride salts that can be metabolized to HCl represent potential HCl. Examples include ammonium chloride (NH_4Cl), lysine HCl, and arginine HCl. The hyperchloremic metabolic acidosis of diarrhea is usually caused by the loss of potential $NaHCO_3$ salts, including sodium acetate and sodium butyrate, into the stool. This is partially responsible for the metabolic acidosis of the patient in Case 11. Other causes of hyperchloremic metabolic acidosis are listed in Table 18.

TABLE 18 Causes of Hyperchloremic (Normal Anion Gap) Metabolic Acidosis

- Gastrointestinal loss of HCO_3
  - Diarrhea
  - Ureterosigmoidostomy
- Renal HCO_3 loss
  - Proximal renal tubular acidosis
    - Isolated — sporadic, familial
    - Fanconi's syndrome — with phosphaturia, glucosuria, uricosuria, aminoaciduria
      - Familial, cystinosis, tyrosinemia, multiple myeloma, Wilson's disease, ifosfamide, osteopetrosis
  - Carbonic anhydrase inhibitors
  - Ileal bladder
- Reduced renal H^+ secretion
  - Distal renal tubular acidosis
    - Familial, hypercalcemic-hypercalciuric states, Sjögren's syndrome, autoimmune diseases, amphotericin B, renal transplant
  - Type 4 renal tubular acidosis
    - Hyporeninemic-hypoaldosterone – diabetes mellitus, tubulointerstitial diseases, NSAIDs
    - Defective mineralocorticoid synthesis or secretion – chronic heparin therapy, Addison's disease, congenital adrenal defects
    - Inadequate renal response to mineralocorticoids – sickle cell disease, systemic lupus erythematosus, potassium-sparing diuretics, "chloride shunts"
  - Early uremia
- HCl/HCl precursor ingestion/infusion
  - HCl
  - NH_4Cl
  - Arginine HCl
- Other
  - Post–chronic hyperventilation
  - Recovery from diabetic ketoacidosis
  - Toluene inhalation

NSAIDs = nonsteroidal anti-inflammatory drugs

All types of renal tubular acidoses (RTA) cause hyperchloremic metabolic acidosis. *Proximal RTA* is caused by a reduced renal $NaHCO_3$ reabsorptive capacity. If the serum [HCO_3] is increased above this abnormally low renal tubule threshold (for example, when exogenous sodium bicarbonate is administered), these patients excrete $NaHCO_3$ in their urine. However, their urine is appropriately acidified when their serum [HCO_3] falls below this threshold level. *Distal RTA* results from an inability of the renal tubules to generate and/or maintain a normal pH gradient (normal minimal urinary pH is < 5.5). Patients with distal RTA will always excrete inappropriately alkaline urine. Distal RTA frequently leads to medullary calcifications and calcium kidney stones (due to hypercalciuria and deficient urinary citrate excretion). The presence of hyperchloremic metabolic acidosis and an alkaline urinary pH suggests the diagnosis of RTA. However, urinary tract infections can also alkalinize the urine because certain bacteria will metabolize urea to ammonium and carbon dioxide. Occasional patients with hyperchloremic metabolic acidosis and marked hypokalemia secondary to diarrhea will excrete alkaline urine because of very high urinary [NH_4]. *Type 4 RTA* is a hyperkalemic, hyperchloremic metabolic acidosis that is usually due to hypoaldosteronism or an inadequate renal tubular response to aldosterone. This leads to hyperkalemia, which inhibits renal NH_4 synthesis and excretion and contributes to the development of metabolic acidosis.

When gastrointestinal epithelium is exposed to urine, it will absorb chloride from, and secrete HCO_3 and potassium into, the urine. This results in hypokalemic, hyperchloremic metabolic acidosis. Ureterosigmoidostomy, ileal loop bladders, or any ileal or colonic segment interposed into the urinary stream can cause this derangement.

Distal RTA can generally be treated with 60 to 100 meq daily of sodium bicarbonate or potential sodium bicarbonate (such as Shohl's solution). Sodium bicarbonate simultaneously corrects the acidosis and volume contraction, ameliorates renal potassium wasting, and increases urinary citrate levels. Increased urinary citrate excretion protects against renal papillary calcification and kidney stone formation. (Bicarbonate therapy is generally not helpful in patients with proximal RTA and may worsen hypokalemia.) The metabolic acidosis and volume depletion produced by diarrhea can also be corrected by the administration of sodium bicarbonate and sodium chloride. These salts should be used to treat the patient in Case 11. The acidosis of type 4 RTA generally improves with correction of hyperkalemia. Some patients with type 4 RTA require exogenous mineralocorticoids, others respond well to diuretics, and still others require exogenous sodium bicarbonate administration. The underlying pathology can sometimes also be corrected (that is, obstructive uropathy).

Metabolic Acidosis with an Increased Anion Gap

Anion gap metabolic acidosis develops when organic and/or nonchloride inorganic acids accumulate at rates that exceed their excretory and/or metabolic removal capacity. The most common causes of high anion gap metabolic acidosis are listed in Table 19. Lactic acidosis is usually due to ischemia resulting from local or systemic underperfusion or overt shock. The patient in Case 11 probably has an element of lactic acidosis caused by volume depletion and hypotension. This is a frequent complication when severe diarrhea causes volume depletion. Many drugs and toxins can also cause lactic acidosis. For example, metformin can cause profound lactic acidosis when high drug levels accumulate in patients with renal insufficiency. A number of inherited and acquired enzyme disorders can also cause lactic acidosis. Ketoacidosis usually develops in patients with diabetes mellitus who have poor glucose control and is often precipitated by the metabolic stress of an intercurrent medical or surgical complication. Ketoacidosis can also occur in malnourished patients with chronic alcoholism. The use of sodium bicarbonate to treat lactic or ketoacidosis is controversial. The elevated anion gap in patients with these disorders represents accumulated potential HCO_3, and correction of the underlying disorder will promote conversion of these anions back to HCO_3. Consequently, a true HCO_3 deficit may not exist. If the HCO_3 concentration is very low and the pH is < 7.1, $NaHCO_3$ may be given.

TABLE 19 Causes of High Anion Gap Metabolic Acidosis

Lactic acidosis
Ketoacidosis
Uremia
Methanol ingestion
Ethylene glycol ingestion
Salicylate poisoning

Methanol ingestion causes a formic acidosis, and ethylene glycol is metabolized to glyoxylate and oxalic acid. The oxalate derived from ethylene glycol precipitates with calcium and is deposited in the brain, lungs, peripheral nerves, and kidneys. Renal failure frequently occurs. A plasma osmolal gap (see preceding section on Electrolytes) and abundant urinary calcium oxalate crystals are important diagnostic clues suggesting ethylene glycol poisoning. The treatment of both methanol and ethylene glycol poisoning requires inhibition of alcohol dehydrogenase. This will block conversion of the ingested compound to organic acids and other toxic metabolites. Inhibition is accomplished by administration of ethanol or fomepizole. Hemodialysis is an effective means to remove the ingested poison and its toxic metabolites and to simultaneously correct the metabolic acidosis and electrolyte abnormalities. The patient in Case 10 (see preceding section on Electrolytes) had ingested one of these poisons. She was initially given $NaHCO_3$ and fomepizole, and hemodialysis was then initiated.

KEY POINTS

- **Determine the osmolal gap when an outpatient presents with an unexplained anion gap acidosis. Check the urine sediment for calcium oxalate crystals, which may indicate ethylene glycol poisoning.**
- **In a patient with anion gap metabolic acidosis, the magnitude of increase in anion gap (Δ gap) should be similar to the fall in $[HCO_3]$ ($\Delta[HCO_3^-]$.**

Metabolic Alkalosis

Case 12

A 36-year-old woman comes to the emergency department because of marked tremulousness and irritability. She denies taking any prescribed medications or use of any other drugs. On physical examination, her blood pressure is 105/75 mm Hg. Blood urea nitrogen is 40 mg/dL, serum creatinine 1.9 mg/dL, sodium 130 meq/L, potassium 3.0 meq/L, chloride 85 meq/L, and bicarbonate 38 meq/L. Arterial blood gas studies (with the patient breathing room air) are pH 7.68, $P\text{CO}_2$ 33 mm Hg, and bicarbonate 38 meq/L. Urinary sodium is 50 meq/L, potassium 30 meq/L, and chloride 2 meq.

Metabolic alkalosis represents a primary increase in [HCO_3]. A compensatory increase in arterial $P\text{CO}_2$ should develop (see Table 17). The patient described in Case 12 has an alkaline arterial pH and an elevated [HCO_3] consistent with metabolic alkalosis. She also has an inappropriately low arterial $P\text{CO}_2$. Therefore, she has both metabolic alkalosis and respiratory alkalosis.

Normal kidneys can rapidly excrete large quantities of $NaHCO_3$. The administration or generation of HCO_3 will rarely increase the [HCO_3] unless certain factors exist that reduce renal $NaHCO_3$ excretion. Always try to understand what has increased the [HCO_3] and also why the kidneys are retaining the [HCO_3]. Renal maintenance of metabolic alkalosis is generally due to reduced renal function and/or stimulation of renal tubule HCO_3 reabsorption. Increased reabsorption is caused by ECF volume contraction, hypokalemia, and/or elevated mineralocorticoid activity.

Gastric fluid contains HCl, NaCl, and water. The external loss of gastric fluid due to vomiting or nasogastric tube suction produces metabolic alkalosis. The key pathophysiologic mechanisms responsible for the development and maintenance of gastric alkalosis are as follows: The stomach secretes HCl and NaCl, which are lost in vomitus. Secretion of HCl causes HCO_3 to enter the ECF, and the plasma [HCO_3] increases. This is the generation phase of the metabolic alkalosis. ECF contraction and Cl depletion simultaneously develop. The renal filtered load of HCO_3 increases, and some $NaHCO_3$ is excreted. The bicarbonaturia partially corrects the alkalosis. However, renal $NaHCO_3$ loss causes additional ECF volume contraction, further reducing the GFR. Renin, angiotensin II, and aldosterone levels all increase. The filtered HCO_3 load falls (GFR reduction), and the $NaHCO_3$ that is filtered is avidly reabsorbed by the proximal and distal tubules. The reabsorption of $NaHCO_3$ in the distal tubule is associated with K secretion. Saline expansion of the ECF will reverse all of the factors that drive HCO_3 reabsorption and rapidly correct the alkalosis. KCl administration is usually also required to correct the K deficit that invariably develops.

Another frequent cause of metabolic alkalosis is administration of thiazide and loop diuretics. These diuretics increase renal excretion of NaCl and water and thereby contract the ECF and activate the renin-angiotensin-aldosterone axis. Persistent distal NaCl delivery, Cl depletion, and aldosterone activity combine to accelerate Na reabsorption and the secretion of protons and K in the distal renal tubules (see Figure 6). This generates hypokalemia and metabolic alkalosis. The metabolic alkalosis is maintained by the combination of hypokalemia, ECF contraction, and the distal renal tubule Na delivery and reabsorption. The volume contraction and hypokalemia increase proximal tubule HCO_3 reabsorption. Thus, the kidney is the site of both HCO_3 generation and maintenance in patients with diuretic-induced metabolic alkalosis. Gastric fluid loss and diuretics probably account for about 90% of cases of metabolic alkalosis.

The metabolic alkaloses can be classified on the basis of the urinary [Cl] (Table 20). ECF contraction should stimulate the kidneys to avidly reabsorb filtered Cl, so that the excreted urinary [Cl] will generally be < 20 meq/L. The metabolic alkaloses listed in the low urinary [Cl] group are also called "chloride sensitive" because administration of NaCl expands the ECF and usually corrects the alkalosis. Patients with metabolic alkalosis and high urinary [Cl] (> 20 meq/L) generally have generation and maintenance mechanisms related to persistent mineralocorticoid stimulation and hypokalemia. ECF expansion and hypertension characterize many of these disorders. This group also includes mineralocorticoid-independent acceleration of distal tubule Na^+ reabsorption (Liddle's syndrome) as well as Bartter's syndrome and Gitelman's syndrome (see below). Generally, infusion of NaCl does not correct metabolic alkaloses in the high-urinary-[Cl] group. Consequently, these disorders are also called the "chloride unresponsive," or "chloride resistant," metabolic alkaloses.

Diuretic-induced metabolic alkalosis requires special consideration in regard to the urinary [Cl]. Soon after ingestion or infusion of a diuretic, the urinary [Cl] will increase above 20 meq/L as a result of the diuretic effect. The urinary [Cl] will then fall below 20 meq/L when the diuretic effect wanes. The generation pathophysiology of diuretic-induced hypokalemic metabolic alkalosis is shown in Figure 6. This alkalosis is classified as a "volume sensitive," or low urinary [Cl], metabolic alkalosis even though the measured urinary [Cl] may be low or high.

Bartter's syndrome and Gitelman's syndrome are high urinary [Cl] metabolic alkaloses. We now know that most patients with these disorders have an inherited defect in one of the renal salt transporters. The affected transporters are the same ones that are inhibited by loop and thiazide diuretics. Consequently, the clinical and chemical abnormalities in these patients are similar to those that develop in patients exposed to a constant infusion of a loop diuretic (Bartter's syndrome) or a thiazide diuretic (Gitelman's syndrome). ECF contraction, high renin and aldosterone levels, and a persistently high urinary [Cl] are characteristic.

The very low urinary [Cl] of the patient in Case 12 strongly suggests vomiting or remote diuretic ingestion. It also suggests that NaCl volume expansion will correct the alkalosis.

TABLE 20 Differential Diagnosis of Metabolic Alkalosis

Low Urinary [Cl] (< 20 meq/L) Chloride Responsive	**High Urinary [Cl] (> 20 meq/L) Chloride Unresponsive**
Diuretics (Remote) ⟷	Diuretics (Recent)
Vomiting/nasogastric tube suction	High blood pressure
Status post chronic hypercarbia	Primary hyperaldosteronism
Chloridorrhea	Cushing's disease
	Ectopic ACTH production
	Exogenous mineralocorticoid production
	Mineralocorticoid-like substances
	Liddle's syndrome
	Low blood pressure
	Bartter's syndrome
	Gitelman's syndrome
	Severe potassium depletion

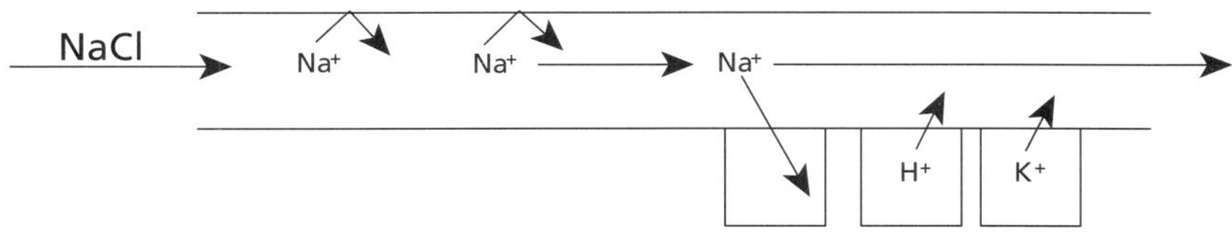

FIGURE 6

Diuretic-induced metabolic alkalosis.
Loop diuretics will reduce Na and Cl reabsorption in the thick ascending limb of Henle and thiazide diuretics reduce Na and Cl reabsorption at more distal sites (the diluting segment). Both diuretics cause increased delivery of Na and Cl to the collecting tubules where Na reabsorption increases H and K secretion.

Respiratory Acidosis

Respiratory acidosis is due to a primary increase in arterial $P\text{CO}_2$. The most common causes are shown in Table 21. The acidemia produced by the high arterial $P\text{CO}_2$ is compensated by an increase in [HCO_3]. Acute respiratory acidosis causes a small increase in [HCO_3] as a result of cellular buffering. Chronic respiratory acidosis causes a larger increase in [HCO_3] by stimulating renal generation of HCO_3. The expected level of compensation is shown in Table 17. Fully compensated chronic respiratory acidosis results in an arterial pH that is slightly below normal. If the increase in [HCO_3] is so great that it results in a normal pH, the [HCO_3] is probably too high, and metabolic alkalosis probably coexists.

KEY POINT

- **Try to identify the source of bicarbonate generation, or administration, and the reason for renal bicarbonate retention in every patient with metabolic alkalosis.**

Respiratory Alkalosis

Hyperventilation reduces the arterial $P\text{CO}_2$, which increases the pH. The causes of respiratory alkalosis are shown in Table 22. The expected compensatory responses for acute and chronic respiratory alkalosis are shown in Table 17.

TABLE 21 Causes of Respiratory Acidosis

Central nervous system depression
- Sedatives
- Central nervous system lesions

Neuromuscular disorders
- Myopathies
- Neuropathies

Thoracic cage restriction
- Kyphoscoliosis
- Scleroderma

Impaired lung motion
- Pleural effusion
- Pneumothorax

Acute obstructive pulmonary disease
- Aspiration
- Tumor
- Bronchospasm

Chronic obstructive pulmonary disease

Miscellaneous
- Ventilator malfunction
- Cardiopulmonary resuscitation

Mixed Acid-Base Disorders

Case 13

A 53-year-old man with a history of chronic alcoholism is hospitalized because of decompensated cirrhosis and probable hepatorenal syndrome. Results of his laboratory studies are shown in Figure 7. Six months ago, his electrolytes were normal (panel 1). On admission, he developed an anion gap metabolic acidosis (panel 2); there is no osmolal gap. Uremic acidosis and lactic acidosis are considered. Following admission, a nasogastric tube is placed. He then develops the electrolyte pattern shown in panel 3. The anion gap remains large, but the [HCO_3] has increased and the [Cl] has decreased. This reflects the combination of still present anion gap metabolic acidosis and superimposed "gastric" metabolic alkalosis. Arterial blood gas studies show that he actually has a triple disturbance because his arterial $P\text{CO}_2$ is too low for his [HCO_3].

Mixed acid-base disorders may cause extreme pH abnormalities (metabolic and respiratory acidosis or metabolic and respiratory alkalosis) or can result in a normal pH (respiratory acidosis and metabolic alkalosis, metabolic acidosis and metabolic alkalosis, etc.). Certain clinical disorders (cardiac arrest, septic shock, drug intoxication, various poisonings, and renal, respiratory, and hepatic failure) are often associated with mixed acid-base disorders (Narins and Emmett, Emmett and Seldin).

Some mixed disorders are due to either inadequate or excessive compensation for a primary acid-base disturbance. For example, when metabolic acidosis reduces the [HCO_3] but the arterial $P\text{CO}_2$ is higher than predicted (see Table 17), respiratory acidosis may coexist. This can result in a very low pH. Mixed

Narins RG, Emmett M. Simple and mixed acid-base disorders: a practical approach. Medicine (Baltimore). 1980;59:161-87. UI: 81011380

Emmett M, Seldin DW. Evaluation of acid-base disorders from plasma composition. In: Seldin DW, Giebisch G, eds. The Regulation of Acid-Base Balance. New York: Raven Press; 1989:213-63.

TABLE 22 Causes of Respiratory Alkalosis

- Anxiety
- Central nervous system disorders
  - Cerebrovascular accident
  - Tumor
  - Infection
- Hormones
  - Progesterone
  - Catecholamines
- Drugs
  - Salicylates
  - Analeptics
- Sepsis and endotoxemia
- Hyperthyroidism
- Hypoxia
- Pregnancy
- Cirrhosis
- Pulmonary edema
- Lung diseases
  - Pulmonary emboli
  - Restrictive lung disorders
  - Pneumonia
- Ventilator-induced

metabolic and respiratory acidosis occurs frequently during cardiopulmonary arrest. If a patient with metabolic acidosis has an arterial P_{CO_2} that is too low, respiratory alkalosis may coexist. This mixed disorder will tend to normalize the pH. Sepsis often causes this particular mixed disorder because endotoxin directly stimulates the respiratory center while hypotension leads to lactic acidosis. Salicylate poisoning also causes mixed metabolic acidosis and respiratory alkalosis because toxic salicylate levels directly stimulate respiration and simultaneously uncouple cellular oxidative metabolism and generate an anion gap acidosis. The patient discussed earlier in Case 12 has a mixed metabolic alkalosis and respiratory alkalosis.

Anion gap metabolic acidosis should increase the anion gap by approximately the same magnitude as the fall in [HCO_3]. When metabolic alkalosis coexists with anion gap metabolic acidosis, the alkalosis will increase the [HCO_3], but the anion gap remains large. When the anion gap is larger than can be explained by the reduction in [HCO_3], mixed metabolic acidosis and metabolic alkalosis are probably present (see Figure 7).

Respiratory alkalosis commonly occurs in patients with severe liver disease as a result of high progesterone levels that stimulate the central nervous system respiratory center and hypoxia related to pulmonary arteriovenous shunts and diaphragms that are "pushed up" by ascites.

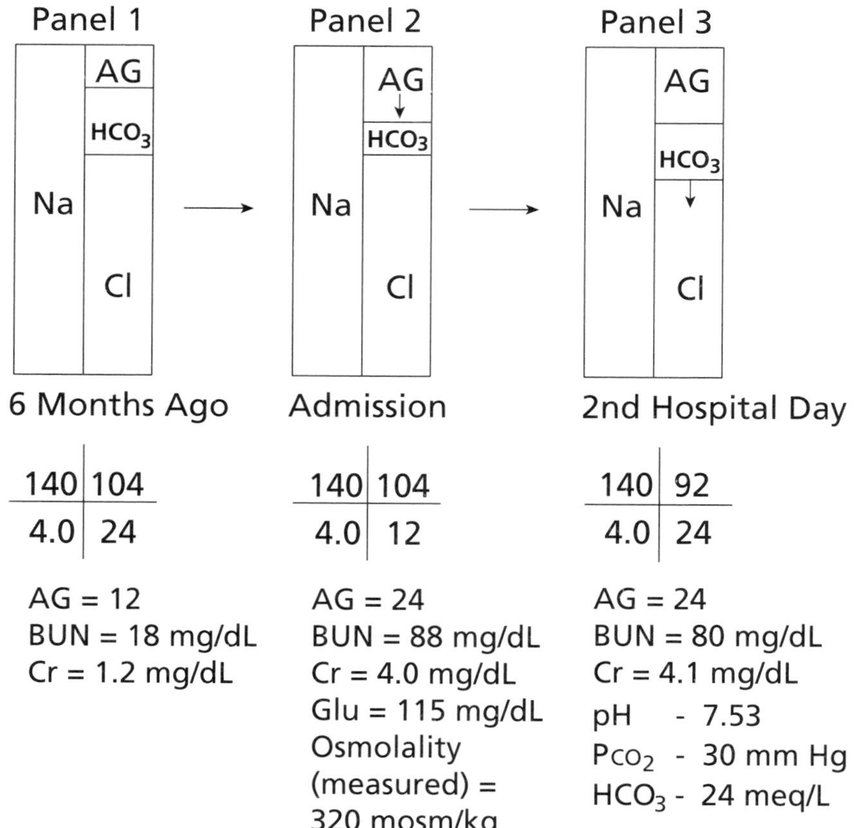

FIGURE 7
Laboratory studies of patient in Case 13.
Unless specified, units are meq/L.
AG = anion gap, BUN = blood urea nitrogen, Cr = serum creatinine, Glu = plasma glucose

Acute Renal Failure

Definition and Causes of Acute Renal Failure

- What is the definition of acute renal failure?
- How often is acute renal failure encountered? What clues does the clinical setting provide?
- What is the most common cause of acute renal failure?
- What are the prognostic implications of acute renal failure in different settings in patients with various diagnoses?

Case 14

A 71-year-old woman is hospitalized after she developed fever, chills, myalgias, nausea, vomiting, and diarrhea 3 days ago and today had dizziness on arising. The patient has had osteoarthritis for 12 years and has been taking sulindac for several years. Her baseline serum creatinine level is 0.7 mg/dL.

On physical examination, she is lethargic but is oriented and arousable. Her pulse rate is 106/min supine and 128/min standing. Blood pressure is 90/70 mm Hg supine, and systolic blood pressure is 60 mm Hg standing. Her chest is clear. There is no cardiac murmur or gallop. Her abdomen is diffusely tender without rebound or rigidity. A stool specimen is trace positive for occult blood. There is no sacral or lower extremity edema.

Blood urea nitrogen is 80 mg/dL, serum creatinine 1.7 mg/dL, sodium 145 meq/L, potassium 3.2 meq/L, chloride 109 meq/L, and bicarbonate 20 meq/L. Urinalysis shows a specific gravity of 1.030, trace protein, trace ketones, and no glucose. Microscopic examination of the urine is normal. Urinary sodium is 8 meq/L, urinary creatinine 63 mg/dL, and urine osmolality 630 mosm/kg H_2O. A 24-hour urine volume measurement, obtained on the first day of admission, is 340 mL.

Acute renal failure (ARF) is defined as a sudden diminution in glomerular filtration rate (GFR). The diagnosis is usually associated with an increasing blood urea nitrogen concentration (azotemia) and increasing serum creatinine concentration. ARF can be diagnosed with certainty when the patient's prior renal function is known and a decrement is documented.

Before considering the diagnosis of intrinsic renal disease, disorders of extracellular fluid (ECF) volume (prerenal azotemia) and obstructive (postrenal) causes of renal insufficiency must be excluded (Figure 8). The evaluation of patients with ARF should include a history of recent medications and procedures and examination of hemodynamic and volume status, urinalysis, and urinary diagnostic indices (Miller et al.). Renal ultrasonography may be useful in assessing the presence of urinary tract obstruction or of chronic renal insufficiency. Renal biopsy may be valuable in those few patients in whom the diagnosis is still unclear.

Miller TR, Anderson RJ, Linas SL, Henrich WL, Berns AS, Gabow PA, et al. Urinary diagnostic indices in acute renal failure. A prospective study. Ann Intern Med. 1978;89:47-50. UI: 78209200

ARF occurs in 2% to 5% of patients in tertiary care centers and in up to one third of patients in intensive care units. It rarely occurs in outpatients. Prerenal azotemia, however, is the most common cause of ARF in both outpatients and hospitalized patients.

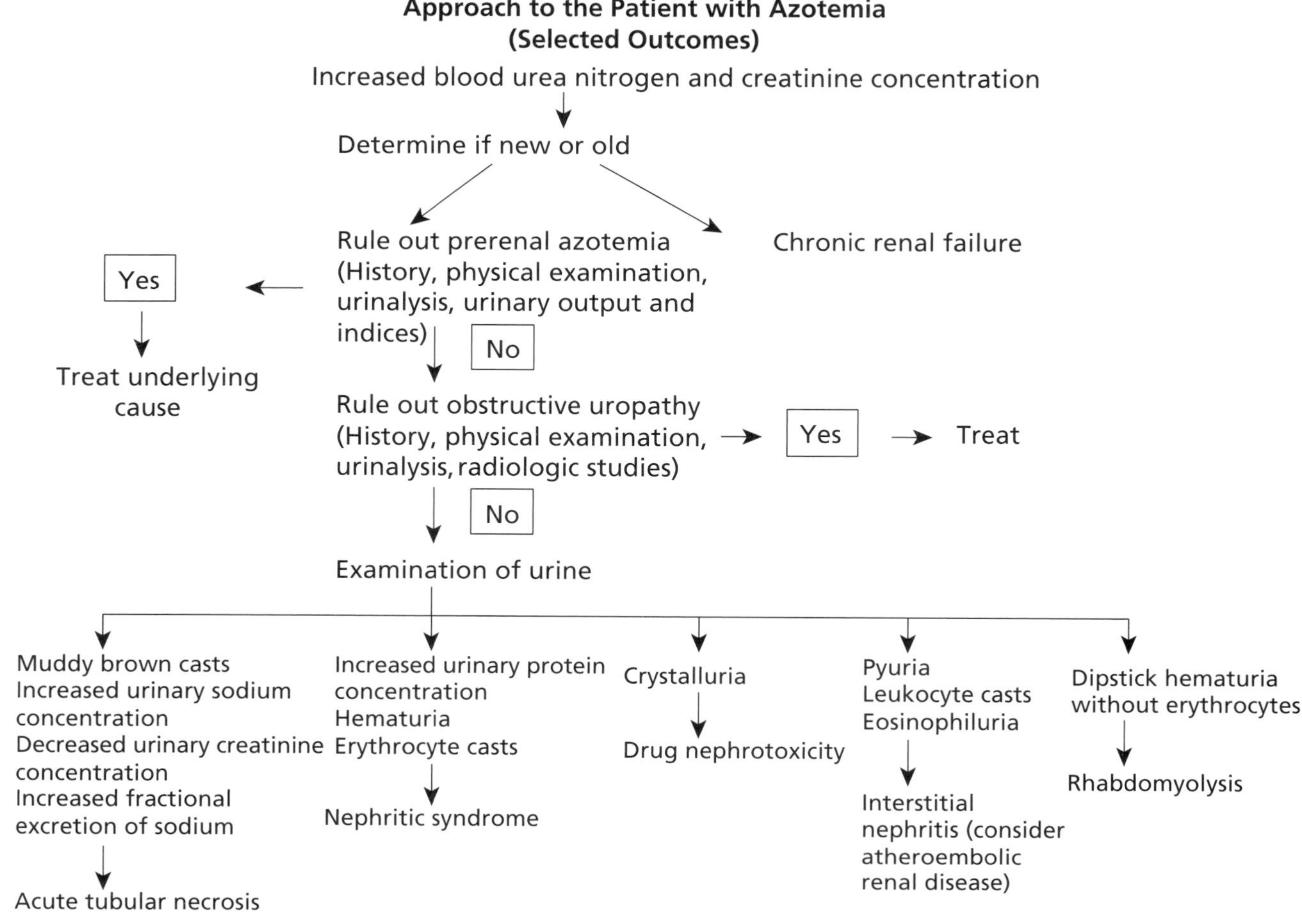

FIGURE 8

Prerenal Azotemia

Prerenal azotemia due to decreased renal perfusion occurs in patients with both volume depletion and volume overload. The most frequent cause of prerenal azotemia is ECF volume depletion. Common causes of volume depletion are shown in Table 23. ECF volume depletion causes stimulation of the sympathetic nervous system and the renin-angiotensin-aldosterone system. This results in increased renal tubular sodium reabsorption in the proximal and distal portions of the nephron and increased release of antidiuretic hormone (ADH), which mediates water reabsorption in the collecting ducts. Therefore, the urine of patients with prerenal azotemia is characterized by low volume, low urinary sodium concentration, increased urinary creatinine concentration, and high osmolality (see Figure 8). Microscopic examination of the urine is generally normal. This is the clinical constellation illustrated by the patient in Case 14.

Fever, surgery, amino acid infusion, increased protein intake or catabolism, and therapy with tetracycline or glucocorticoids increase urea production, which results in azotemia without a decreased GFR or increased serum creatinine concentration. Administration of trimethoprim and cimetidine decreases proximal renal tubular secretion of creatinine and urinary creatinine excretion, thereby increasing circulating serum creatinine levels in the absence of changes in GFR. The use of nonsteroidal anti-inflammatory drugs (NSAIDs) may be

TABLE 23 Causes of Prerenal Azotemia

Volume depletion
- Deficient fluid intake
- Diarrhea
- Nasogastric tube suction
- Vomiting
- Hemorrhage
- Burns

Volume overload — decreased effective arterial blood volume
- Congestive heart failure
- Liver disease with ascites
- Nephrotic syndrome
- Capillary leak syndromes
- Third spacing

Decreased renal perfusion — normal volume status
- Severe hypoalbuminemia
- Sepsis
- Psychotropic drug overdoses
- Excessive antihypertensive treatment resulting in hypotension secondary to peripheral vasodilatation

Drugs interfering with renal blood flow
- Vasoconstrictors
- Pressor agents
- Nonsteroidal anti-inflammatory drugs
- Angiotensin-converting enzyme inhibitors

associated with functional reversible decrements in renal blood flow and GFR as a result of inhibition of renal afferent arteriolar vasodilatation. This is particularly evident in patients with preexisting renal insufficiency or concurrent volume depletion. Hypercalcemia may cause renal vasoconstriction and a decreased GFR but is also associated with renal tubular defects that may cause polyuria, worsening of volume depletion, and increase in serum calcium concentration. This can lead to a vicious circle of volume depletion and increasing hypercalcemia in the absence of intrinsic renal disease.

Patients who have ARF have increased morbidity and a 5- to 15-fold increase in mortality compared with patients who do not have ARF. Patients with prerenal azotemia generally have a favorable prognosis. Recent studies, however, suggest that the mortality rate for patients with prerenal azotemia requiring nephrology consultation or treatment in an intensive care unit may be as high as 20% to 52%, probably because of the severity of the underlying presenting condition.

Determining the fractional excretion of sodium (FE_{Na}) may be useful in patients with oliguria. The FE_{Na} represents the percentage of the total filtered sodium that is ultimately excreted in the final urine. The FE_{Na} can be determined from a spot urine specimen with simultaneous determinations of plasma sodium and creatinine concentrations:

$$FE_{Na} = \frac{\dfrac{\text{Urine Na concentration}}{\text{Plasma Na concentration}}}{\dfrac{\text{Urine creatinine concentration}}{\text{Plasma creatinine concentration}}} \times 100\%$$

KEY POINTS

- Prerenal azotemia is the most common cause of acute renal failure.
- Prerenal azotemia is by far the most common cause of acute renal failure in outpatients.
- In hospitalized patients, prerenal azotemia has an ominous prognosis if it complicates a disease with substantial morbidity.
- Nonsteroidal anti-inflammatory drugs may worsen renal function in patients with volume depletion or volume overload and prerenal azotemia.
- Determination of the FE_{Na} is most useful in patients with oliguria and acute renal failure.

The FE_{Na} is characteristically less than 1% in patients with prerenal azotemia. This is the situation in the patient in Case 14. In patients with ARF, a FE_{Na} greater than 1% usually indicates an intrinsic renal cause of azotemia, but a high value is never normal in patients with oliguria. Diuretic use and osmotic diuresis due to glycosuria in patients with diabetes mellitus may be associated with natriuresis, volume depletion, and subsequent prerenal azotemia. The urinary sodium concentration and FE_{Na} may be high in such patients and therefore may be unreliable indicators of the volume-depleted state during diuresis. Determination of the FE_{Na} is most useful in patients with oliguria and ARF.

Prerenal Azotemia in Patients Treated with Diuretics

- Is the evaluation of FE_{Na} useful in patients who are being treated with diuretics?
- Should diuretics be discontinued in a patient who seems to be resistant to these agents and has developed prerenal azotemia?

Case 15

A 45-year-old man is brought to the emergency department because of increasing edema and dyspnea. He has a history of congestive heart failure due to alcoholic cardiomyopathy. He stopped drinking alcohol for several months and was treated with digoxin and furosemide, but his dyspnea increased and was associated with new-onset orthopnea and pedal edema. The dose of furosemide was increased, and he improved transiently. He then noted increasing edema and dyspnea, and the dose of furosemide was increased once again. However, he continued to feel uncomfortable and is evaluated in the emergency department.

On physical examination, his pulse rate is 112/min and regular, and blood pressure is 100/72 mm Hg. Neck veins are distended 3 cm at 45 degrees, and hepatojugular reflux is present. Bilateral crackles are heard, and an S_3 gallop is auscultated. There is bilateral lower extremity edema. The patient is hospitalized.

Blood urea nitrogen on admission is 80 mg/dL, serum creatinine 4.0 mg/dL, sodium 130 meq/L, potassium 3.2 meq/L, chloride 99 meq/L, and bicarbonate 20 meq/L. Urinalysis shows a specific gravity of 1.012, trace protein, trace ketones, and no glucose. Microscopic examination is normal. Urinary sodium concentration is 48 meq/L, and urine osmolality is 330 mosm/kg H_2O. FE_{Na} is 4.5%. A 24-hour urine volume determination is 260 mL on the first hospital day, although the patient is being treated with high-dose intravenous furosemide.

Patients with decreased renal blood flow despite clinical volume overload (such as patients with congestive heart failure, other cardiovascular diseases, or ascites) have renal responses similar to those encountered in patients with volume depletion (see Table 23). Findings on urinalysis and microscopic examination are also similar to findings in patients with volume depletion. Treatment consists of normalizing the ECF volume and treating the underlying disease with diuretics, if possible (Kramer et al.). FE_{Na} may still be a useful measure in patients with ARF who are treated with diuretics, since a low value substantiates the diagnosis of prerenal azotemia and suggests resistance to diuretic action. A high FE_{Na} alone cannot distinguish an intrinsic renal cause of azotemia from prerenal azotemia in a patient treated with diuretics.

Kramer BK, Schweda F, Riegger GA. Diuretic treatment and diuretic resistance in heart failure. Am J Med. 1999;106:90-6. UI: 99251841

KEY POINTS

- Prerenal azotemia may develop in patients with volume overload as well as in patients with volume depletion.
- A FE_{Na} greater than 1% is never physiologic in patients with oliguria.

Prerenal Azotemia in Patients Treated with Angiotensin-Converting Enzyme Inhibitors

- When do angiotensin-converting enzyme inhibitors cause acute renal failure?
- What is the hemodynamic cause of acute renal failure in such patients?

Patients with decreased renal blood flow secondary to various forms of renal vascular disease (such as renal artery stenosis, renal artery thrombosis, and renal embolic disease) may have decreased renal perfusion. The use of angiotensin-converting enzyme (ACE) inhibitors may also be associated with functional reversible decrements in renal blood flow and GFR, particularly in patients with preexisting renal insufficiency, renal vascular disease, or concurrent volume depletion. ACE inhibitors decrease resistance of the postglomerular efferent arterioles and decrease net glomerular filtration pressure. This causes a decreased GFR in patients with renal insufficiency or renal artery stenosis. A net decrease in glomerular filtration pressure results, especially in patients with preexisting volume depletion or renal insufficiency. Similar hemodynamic responses may occur in patients being treated with angiotensin II receptor blockers.

KEY POINTS

- Prerenal azotemia may be encountered in patients with volume overload or volume depletion who are being treated with ACE inhibitors or angiotensin II receptor blockers.
- Patients with a decrement in renal function after treatment with ACE inhibitors or angiotensin II receptor blockers should be screened for the presence of a solitary kidney or renal vascular disease.
- The acute renal failure associated with administration of ACE inhibitors or angiotensin II receptor blockers is a result of disordered hemodynamics that initiates a type of prerenal azotemia.
- Azotemia is frequently reversible after discontinuation of the drug.

Treatment of Prerenal Azotemia

Initial treatment of prerenal azotemia consists of optimizing volume status. Patients with volume depletion should be treated with intravenous normal saline and should be carefully observed for changes in volume status and urine flow. Prerenal azotemia and oliguria are typically reversed after fluid administration. The most appropriate management of patients with congestive heart failure or ascites is treatment of the underlying disease, use of inotropic drugs to improve cardiac output, and normalization of ECF volume (frequently with diuretics) to improve cardiac output and renal perfusion. In a patient in whom drug effects are suspected as causing the prerenal azotemia, the drug in question should be discontinued, and the patient's clinical course should be observed. Patients with hypercalcemia should be treated with volume repletion and a loop diuretic, such as furosemide, to maximize urinary calcium excretion.

Postrenal Azotemia (Urinary Tract Obstruction)

- What are the causes of postrenal azotemia?
- How should patients with postrenal azotemia be treated?
- What is the outcome for patients with postrenal azotemia?

Obstruction of the urinary outflow tract may also cause ARF (see Figure 8). To cause azotemia, obstruction must involve the outflow tracts of two normal kidneys or of one kidney if bilateral renal dysfunction previously occurred. The diagnosis of acute or chronic urinary tract obstruction should be considered strongly in patients who have had abdominal or pelvic surgery, gynecologic or prostate gland neoplasms, or radiation therapy. Patients who develop chronic urinary tract obstruction are often asymptomatic. Although the presence of anuria suggests complete obstruction, urinary frequency, polyuria, oliguria, and nocturia may often accompany partial urinary tract obstruction. Urine indices and urinary sodium concentration are not reliable findings in patients with urinary tract obstruction. The ratio of blood urea nitrogen to serum creatinine may be elevated as a result of decreased tubular flow and enhanced tubular urea reabsorption.

Demonstration of hydronephrosis by ultrasonography is sensitive and specific in confirming the diagnosis of urinary tract obstruction. If periureteral metastatic disease or retroperitoneal fibrosis encases the ureters or if the results

KEY POINTS

- Ultrasonography is the first step in the evaluation of patients with suspected urinary tract obstruction.
- Postobstructive diuresis is relatively uncommon and is usually self-limited.
- Postobstructive diuresis must be distinguished from a physiologic response to relief of obstruction.
- Determination of the FE_{Na} is rarely useful in the diagnosis of patients with urinary tract obstruction.
- Urinary solute excretion rates help to delineate the amount of fluid repletion needed after correction of the urinary tract obstruction.
- The outcome in patients with urinary tract obstruction depends on prompt recognition and treatment and on the patient's underlying illness.

of the ultrasound examination are equivocal, CT or MRI may provide better diagnostic discrimination. Antegrade or retrograde intravenous pyelography or percutaneous nephrostomy is only rarely used to diagnose urinary tract obstruction.

Polyuria may occur as a physiologic response after correction of a urinary tract obstruction, or postobstructive diuresis may occur because of sodium and water retention and abnormal renal tubular handling of sodium and water. An appropriate physiologic diuresis must be distinguished from the infrequent pathologic diuresis, which is manifested by signs of volume depletion, hypotension, and possibly by recurrent azotemia. Serum and urinary electrolyte concentrations and clinical and laboratory determinations of volume status provide a rational basis for fluid replacement. Both the duration and the severity of obstruction are important factors associated with recovery of renal function. Complete return to baseline function is possible if the obstruction is partial or of relatively short duration, although tubular defects may persist for some time. Limited recovery may be expected when high-grade urinary tract obstruction exceeds 3 months. Patient survival depends on the severity of the underlying illness. Mortality rates are highest in patients with malignancy.

Intrinsic Acute Renal Failure

- What is the most common cause of intrinsic acute renal failure in hospitalized patients?
- Does the clinical setting provide clues to the diagnosis and prognosis in patients with intrinsic acute renal failure?

Case 16

A 70-year-old man with coronary artery disease and atherosclerotic peripheral vascular disease is hospitalized because of abdominal pain. He has had hypertension for 20 years and hypercholesterolemia for 8 years, both of which are well controlled by various medications.

On physical examination, his pulse rate is 112/min and regular, and blood pressure is 90/64 mm Hg. His chest is clear. No cardiac murmurs or gallops are heard. His abdomen is diffusely tender. There is trace bilateral lower extremity edema. Rectal examination shows a boggy but normal-sized prostate gland, good tone, and a stool specimen that is positive for occult blood. Blood urea nitrogen is 29 mg/dL, and serum creatinine is 1.4 mg/dL. Urinalysis shows a specific gravity of 1.018, trace protein, and no glucose or ketones. Urinary sodium concentration is 60 meq/L. Microscopic examination of the urine is normal.

The patient undergoes emergency arteriography for intestinal ischemia and subsequently has a right hemicolectomy. On the first postoperative day, he develops fever, and cefotaxime and tobramycin are begun. On the second postoperative day, his blood pressure is 130/80 mm Hg, but 12-hour urine output is 135 mL. Blood urea nitrogen is 68 mg/dL, and serum creatinine is 4.1 mg/dL. Urinalysis reveals a specific gravity of 1.009. Microscopic examination shows granular casts.

Acute tubular necrosis is common in patients in intensive care units and is the most frequent cause of ARF due to intrinsic renal disease in hospitalized patients. The pathogenesis is usually associated with renal ischemia and/or toxicity. The decreased GFR has been ascribed to vasoconstriction, intratubular obstruction secondary to swollen necrotic cells, backleak of glomerular filtrate through disrupted proximal tubules, and decreased glomerular permeability.

Most patients with acute tubular necrosis have multiple associated conditions, such as hypotension, sepsis, or the administration of nephrotoxic agents. Development of renal insufficiency may be insidious or acute. Because of the hyperbolic relationship between the serum creatinine concentration and the GFR, a patient with early-stage acute tubular necrosis who has relatively little muscle mass may lose as much as 50% of renal function, but the increasing serum creatinine concentration may still be in the normal range. Patients with acute tubular necrosis typically have an initial oliguric phase that is variable in degree and duration (Klahr and Miller). The oliguric phase may be so brief as to be clinically inapparent, or it may continue for as long as 10 to 14 days. Occasionally, oliguria will be irreversible, and chronic renal failure or end-stage renal disease will result. More often, the oliguric phase is followed by a diuretic phase, which is sometimes characterized by large increases in urine flow. The diuresis is a consequence of the increasing GFR coupled with the inability of regenerating tubules to reabsorb sodium and water normally. Fluid and electrolyte disorders such as volume depletion, hyponatremia, or hypernatremia may result. If recovery occurs, the long-term prognosis is good, but abnormal renal function is often present and may persist for years.

Klahr S, Miller SB. Acute oliguria. N Engl J Med. 1998;338:671-5. UI: 98135523

Patients with acute tubular necrosis typically have abnormal urine with pigmented tubular epithelial cell casts and debris. The urinary sodium concentration and FE_{Na} are usually high, whereas the urine osmolality is not increased compared with the plasma osmolality. The latter reflects the inability of the tubules to reabsorb sodium and water. The urinary creatinine concentration is typically low, reflecting both the diminution in GFR and the reabsorption of tubular fluid (see Figure 8). In patients with nonoliguric ARF, however, urinary diagnostic indices are unreliable and should not be used.

KEY POINTS

- Acute tubular necrosis is a common cause of acute renal failure in patients in intensive care units.
- The pathogenesis of acute tubular necrosis usually involves multiple mechanisms.
- In addition to renal ischemia, a toxic insult is usually implicated in the pathogenesis of acute tubular necrosis.
- Urinalysis is useful in making the diagnosis; urinary indices are most sensitive in patients with oliguria.
- Patients with acute tubular necrosis typically have an oliguric phase, followed by a diuretic phase.

Management of Intrinsic Acute Renal Failure

- What is the prognosis for hospitalized patients with acute renal failure due to acute tubular necrosis?
- What therapy provides the best outcome in hospitalized patients with acute renal failure due to acute tubular necrosis?
- When in the course of the disease should renal replacement therapy be started?
- How are the amount and duration of renal replacement therapy determined?
- Are there advantages of one modality of renal replacement therapy compared with another?
- Can pharmacologic therapy improve outcome in patients with acute renal failure?

After establishing the diagnosis of ARF related to intrinsic renal disease, the clinician must attempt to minimize renal parenchymal injury, prevent symptoms of uremia, ensure metabolic balance, and promote recovery of renal function (Star; Vijayan and Miller). Optimizing the patient's clinical volume status is imperative. Sodium and water restriction may be necessary, especially in patients with oliguria and ARF. Protein restriction, administration of essential amino acids, and maintenance of carbohydrate intake may limit catabolism but maintain nitrogen balance. Potassium and phosphorus intake should be restricted. Hyperkalemia and acidemia should be identified and treated. Magnesium-containing antacids and medications that can reduce the GFR or interfere with potassium disposition should be discontinued. Medications should be adjusted according to the patient's degree of renal insufficiency.

Star RA. Treatment of acute renal failure. Kidney Int. 1998;54:1817-31. UI: 99070358

Vijayan A, Miller SB. Acute renal failure: prevention and nondialytic therapy. Semin Nephrol. 1998:18:523-32. UI: 9842556

Diuretics, often in high doses, have been advocated for the treatment of oliguric acute tubular necrosis; however, there are no rigorously controlled clinical trials that demonstrate the efficacy of diuretic agents in modifying the course or outcome of this disorder. Mannitol, furosemide, and ethacrynic acid have been used with variable success. High-dose mannitol must be administered cautiously in patients with oliguric ARF, since mannitol-induced hyperosmolarity may cause ECF volume expansion and hyperkalemia.

Hemodialysis, peritoneal dialysis, continuous arteriovenous hemofiltration (CAVH), and continuous venovenous hemofiltration (CVVH) may be necessary for the treatment of complications of ARF. Each has specific advantages and disadvantages (Conger). Some indications for emergent dialysis in patients with ARF are hyperkalemia, acidemia, and hypoxemia from volume overload that is refractory to treatment. Hemodialysis also provides rapid systemic treatment of hyperkalemia and volume overload, but the procedure is ultimately limited by the patient's mean arterial pressure and cardiovascular status (Evanson et al.). Hemodialysis also requires systemic anticoagulation and access to the circulation through relatively large blood vessels. Peritoneal dialysis is easily initiated, is useful in the hemodynamically unstable patient, and does not require systemic anticoagulation. Peritoneal dialysis may be less useful than hemodialysis in the emergent treatment of hyperkalemia or acidemia; however, it provides good long-term control of fluid balance. Peritoneal dialysis is relatively contraindicated in patients who have recently undergone abdominal surgery.

Conger J. Dialysis and related therapies. Semin Nephrol. 1998;18:533-40. UI: 98425577

Evanson JA, Himmelfarb J, Wingard R, Knights S, Shyr Y, Schulman G, et al. Prescribed versus delivered dialysis in acute renal failure. Am J Kidney Dis. 1998; 32:731-8. UI: 99036327

CAVH and CVVH are useful in hemodynamically unstable patients with hypotension. Both CAVH and CVVH provide excellent fluid control and allow the administration of large amounts of fluid, particularly for total parenteral nutrition. However, these continuous therapeutic procedures are relatively inefficient in treating patients with uremia and its complications. The clearance of uremic toxins may be enhanced by adding a dialytic component (continuous arteriovenous hemodiafiltration or continuous venovenous hemodiafiltration). Continuous filtration procedures have been advocated to clear vasoactive substances such as cytokines in patients with sepsis and multi-organ system failure. However, well-designed, prospective, controlled clinical trials of different types of continuous and intermittent renal replacement procedures for patients with ARF have not yielded conclusive data supporting the use of a particular procedure.

The mortality rate in patients with ARF has been relatively unchanged over the past four decades and has been as high as 80% in studies of patients in intensive care units. These findings may reflect the growth of an aging population with preexisting chronic illnesses. Hospitalized surgical patients, patients in intensive care units who develop ARF, and patients with oliguria have consistently poorer survival than outpatients, hospitalized medical patients, patients treated in less intensive care settings, and patients with nonoliguric ARF. Up to 15% of patients who undergo cardiac surgery may develop ARF, with a 13% mortality rate. Survival may be as high as 32% in patients with ARF who are being treated with continuous renal replacement therapy in intensive care units. Higher mortality rates occur in the elderly and in patients with more severe oliguric ARF, preexisting chronic disease, respiratory failure requiring mechanical ventilation, multi-organ system failure, jaundice or hepatic failure, neoplasms, hypotension, and coma. The mortality due to ARF is related to the severity of the underlying illness and the patient's previous health status, as measured by several scoring systems. A few surviving patients will require chronic renal replacement therapy (Liano and Pascual).

KEY POINTS

- The mortality from acute renal failure is primarily related to the severity of the underlying illness and is increased in elderly patients, surgical patients, patients in intensive care units, and patients with:
  - Preexisting chronic disease
  - Hypotension
  - Oliguria
  - Respiratory failure requiring mechanical ventilation
  - Multi-organ system failure
  - Jaundice or hepatic failure
  - Neoplasms
  - Coma
- The efficacy of biologic therapies to ameliorate the course of acute renal failure has not yet been documented.
- The type of membrane used for dialysis may confer an advantage in patients with acute renal failure.
- Continuous renal replacement therapies are now used almost as often as peritoneal dialysis and hemodialysis in patients with acute renal failure who are in intensive care units, but this issue remains controversial.
- Therapeutic strategies, including treatment modalities and parameters for solute and fluid clearance, that meaningfully affect outcomes in patients with acute renal failure have not yet been demonstrated.

Liano F, Pascual J. Outcomes in acute renal failure. Semin Nephrol. 1998;18:541-50. UI: 98425578

Conservative management of the complications of ARF is easier in patients with nonoliguric ARF because of their high urine output and their less frequent need for dialysis. Prospective studies of patients with ARF who were treated with polymethylmethacrylate or polyacrylonitrile "biocompatible" dialysis membranes showed improved survival and a reduced course of renal insufficiency compared with patients who were treated with standard cuprophane membranes. For unknown reasons, more recent studies have not confirmed this effect (Jorres et al.). These studies, however, did not control for indications for dialysis or for the amount of dialysis delivered. A recent study linked higher ultrafiltration rates (perhaps associated with increased clearance) with increased survival of patients with ARF who were treated with continuous renal replacement therapy (Ronco et al.). There are currently a paucity of studies to guide the provision, delivery, and timing of fluid and solute removal by intermittent and continuous techniques. The optimal dose of dialysis and target levels of urea to be maintained to optimize outcomes are unknown. Delivered urea clearance is often lower than prescribed because of technical difficulties. The role of parenteral hyperalimentation in improving outcomes in patients with ARF has not been conclusively determined.

In patients with established ARF, the therapeutic effects of vasodilators (including calcium channel blockers), atrial natriuretic peptide, and growth factors are also inconclusive. No study has shown convincing evidence that administration of dopamine results in enhanced clinically significant outcomes in patients with ARF. Patients who underwent suprarenal aortic or renal artery surgery and who were treated with subcutaneous insulin-like growth factor I (IGF-I) had improved maintenance of renal function compared with untreated control patients. Differences were minor, however, and none of the patients enrolled in the study developed ARF (Franklin et al.). In a larger study of patients with established ARF, IGF-I was not effective in improving GFR, serum creatinine concentration, urine output, or mortality (Hirschberg et al.). In another large study, the atrial natriuretic peptide, anaritide, was ineffective in improving dialysis-free survival, except in patients with oliguric ARF (Lewis et al.). Moreover, more recent studies did not show that atrial natriuretic peptide improved the course of patients with oliguric ARF. The use of these agents therefore cannot be recommended.

Jorres A, Gahl GM, Dobis C, Palenakovic MH, Cakalaroski K, Rutkowski B, et al. Hemodialysis-membrane biocompatibility and mortality of patients with dialysis-dependent acute renal failure: a prospective randomised multicentre trial. International Multicentre Study Group. Lancet. 1999;354:1337-41. UI: 20001429

Ronco C, Bellomo R, Homel P, Brendolan A, Dan M, Piccinni P, La Greca G. Effects of different doses in continuous veno-venous haemofiltration on outcomes of acute renal failure: a prospective randomised trial. Lancet. 2000;356:26-30. UI: 20348850

Franklin SC, Moulton M, Sicard GA, Hammerman MR, Miller SB. Insulin-like growth factor I preserves renal function postoperatively. Am J Physiol. 1997;272:F257-9. UI: 97222284

Hirschberg R, Kopple J, Lipsett P, Benjamin E, Minei J, Albertson T, et al. Multicenter clinical trial of recombinant human insulin-like growth factor I in patients with acute renal failure. Kidney Int. 1999;55:2423-32. UI: 99283013

Lewis J, Salem MM, Chertow GM, Weisberg LS, McGrew F, Marbury TC, et al. Atrial natriuretic factor in oliguric acute renal failure. Anaritide Acute Renal Failure Study Group. Am J Kidney Dis. 2000;36:767-74. UI: 20465399

Contrast-Mediated Nephropathy

- What are the most common risk factors for the development of contrast-mediated nephropathy?
- What therapeutic strategies may be used to limit the development of contrast-mediated nephropathy?

The overall incidence of contrast-mediated nephropathy is low but may be markedly increased in high-risk patients with diabetes mellitus and/or renal insufficiency. Contrast-mediated nephropathy typically causes an increased serum creatinine concentration 24 to 48 hours after exposure. The serum creatinine concentration peaks at 3 to 5 days. Contrast-mediated nephropathy comprises a range of disorders from inconsequential enzymuria or slight transient decrease in the GFR to severe irreversible oliguric ARF. Renal function usually returns to baseline in 10 to 14 days. However, renal impairment may be prolonged and may require temporary or, rarely, permanent dialysis. Renal dysfunction is usually not associated with oliguria. Urinalysis typically shows only casts and is nondiagnostic. In patients with contrast-mediated nephropathy, the urine osmolality is usually high and the FE_{Na} is often low, unlike the findings in patients with ARF due to most other causes. Contrast-mediated nephropathy generally is associated with low morbidity and mortality.

Several pathogenic mechanisms for the development of contrast-mediated nephropathy have been proposed, including roles for vasoactive substances such as endothelin, nitric oxide, free oxygen radicals, and adenosine (Solomon). Renal hemodynamic changes following exposure to contrast agents include an initial brief period of vasodilatation followed by a more prolonged period of

Solomon R. Radiocontrast-induced nephropathy. Semin Nephrol. 1998;18:551-7. UI: 98425579

KEY POINTS

- **Approaches to decreasing the incidence of contrast-mediated nephropathy in patients with renal insufficiency include:**
  - **Performing procedures in carefully selected patients using the minimum amount of contrast agent.**
  - **Ensuring optimal fluid balance.**
  - **Discontinuing concurrent administration of nephrotoxic medications, if possible.**
  - **Administering half-normal saline before the procedure.**
- **Oral acetylcysteine may be a promising addition to the therapeutic armamentarium for decreasing the incidence of contrast-mediated nephropathy in patients with chronic renal insufficiency.**

vasoconstriction that results in diminished renal blood flow and GFR. For unknown reasons, patients with diabetes mellitus have a paradoxical vasodilatory response to contrast agents.

Prevention of contrast-mediated nephropathy is best accomplished by avoiding administration of contrast agents in high-risk patients and by choosing alternative diagnostic procedures such as radionuclide or MRI scans and ultrasonography if possible. Potentially nephrotoxic drugs should be discontinued in patients with renal insufficiency who are receiving contrast agents. The use of nonionic, less hyperosmolar agents such as metrizamide may decrease the incidence of contrast-mediated nephropathy in patients with renal insufficiency, regardless of whether these patients have diabetes mellitus. The cost of such agents, however, may be substantial. In relatively low-risk patient populations, use of nonionic agents is not associated with a reduced incidence of contrast-mediated nephropathy. In high-risk patients, limiting the dose of the contrast agent and providing volume expansion with 5% dextrose/half-normal saline before the procedure decrease the incidence of nephropathy. Although other approaches to decreasing contrast-mediated nephropathy have been studied (for example, administration of calcium channel blockers and theophylline or the use of dialysis to remove contrast agents in patients with advanced renal dysfunction or diabetes mellitus), their role has not been rigorously defined nor has their superiority to administration of half-normal saline been shown. Recently, oral administration of acetylcysteine in addition to half-normal saline was associated with a decrease in the proportion of patients with chronic renal insufficiency who developed contrast-mediated nephropathy (Tepel et al.). The population that will benefit most from this intervention remains to be determined.

Tepel M, van der Geit M, Schwarzfeld C, Laufer U, Liermann D, Zidek W. Prevention of radiographic-contrast-agent-induced reductions in renal function by acetylcysteine. N Engl J Med. 2000;343:210-2. UI: 20344355

Antibiotic-Induced Nephrotoxicity

- What drugs are commonly associated with nephrotoxic ARF in patients who are being treated for infection?
- How does nephrotoxic renal disease differ from acute tubular necrosis?
- How does nephrotoxic renal disease differ from acute interstitial nephritis?
- What are the most common risk factors for the development of renal insufficiency?
- Does the clinical setting provide clues to the diagnosis?
- What therapeutic strategies may be used to limit the development of nephrotoxicity?

Nephrotoxic drugs, often antibiotics, are typically eliminated by the kidneys and tend to accumulate when the GFR is decreased. In contrast to the explosive course of acute tubular necrosis caused by multiple factors in the intensive care unit, the development of nephrotoxicity due to a drug alone is often insidious and occurs more commonly in settings outside the intensive care unit. Seven percent to 29% of hospital-acquired ARF is related to the use of aminoglycoside antibiotics. The risk of nephrotoxicity due to aminoglycoside antibiotics increases with increasing patient age, duration of therapy, presence of volume depletion or hypotension, and preexisting renal disease. In a recent study, 15% of elderly patients treated with aminoglycoside antibiotics developed nephrotoxicity; the incidence increased markedly after 1 week of therapy (Paterson et al.). Aminoglycoside antibiotic nephrotoxicity is associated with relatively low mortality rates but does increases hospitalization costs.

Paterson DL, Robson JMB, Wagener MM. Risk factors for toxicity in elderly patients given aminoglycosides once daily. J Gen Intern Med. 1998;13:735-9. UI: 99047003

Aminoglycoside antibiotic nephrotoxicity may be associated with renal potassium and magnesium wasting, resulting in the development of hypokalemia, hypomagnesemia, and hypocalcemia. Polyuria and nephrogenic diabetes insipidus may result. Many patients who are treated with aminoglycoside antibiotics have other risk factors for developing ARF. When aminoglycoside antibiotic nephrotoxicity is the only cause of renal dysfunction, ARF is usually nonoliguric. A decreased GFR may not become clinically apparent until 1 to 2 weeks after initiating therapy. Urinary sodium concentration and FE_{Na} are typically high. In patients with multiple risk factors, the time course for developing ARF may be much shorter.

Because the therapeutic:toxic ratio for aminoglycoside antibiotics is low, monitoring serum peak and trough drug levels is advised. Avoidance of peak and trough gentamicin and tobramycin concentrations greater than 10 μg/mL and 2 μg/mL, respectively, is associated with a lower incidence of nephrotoxicity. Maintenance of volume status and repletion of electrolytes are important for patients who are treated with aminoglycoside antibiotics. If ARF develops, the drug should be discontinued if clinically feasible. However, renal failure may progress even after discontinuation of the antibiotic or reduction in its dose. If the drug must be continued throughout the course of renal insufficiency, the antibiotic serum concentration is a reliable guide to determining the dose. Once-daily aminoglycoside antibiotic administration has been advocated to reduce the incidence of nephrotoxicity, but such regimens have not been shown unequivocally to improve outcomes. The duration of therapy may be an important risk factor for the development of nephrotoxicity in elderly patients treated with once-daily aminoglycoside antibiotics.

Irreversible nephrotoxicity due to amphotericin B is related to the total cumulative dose administered and rarely develops unless the total dose exceeds 2 g. Amphotericin B reacts with cell membrane sterols, causing renal vasoconstriction and renal arteriolar and tubular structural damage. Elderly and volume-depleted patients are at greatest risk. Volume repletion and use of lipid-complexed preparations may reduce toxicity. ARF is usually nonoliguric and is slowly progressive but causes little proteinuria. Tubular disorders such as distal renal tubular acidosis and abnormal water and cation reabsorption may be noted. Newer antifungal preparations may be less toxic than amphotericin B.

Pentamidine and vancomycin may also cause nephrotoxicity. Pentamidine is concentrated in renal tissue but is poorly cleared by the kidneys. Parenteral administration of pentamidine has been associated with ARF in 25% to 73% of treated patients. The aerosolized preparation is only rarely associated with ARF. Vancomycin is excreted primarily by the kidneys. If used alone, nephrotoxicity occurs infrequently, but vancomycin may potentiate aminoglycoside antibiotic nephrotoxicity. Finally, Chinese herbs and other alternative therapeutics may cause ARF in outpatients. Clinicians should be aware of the nephrotoxic effects of these preparations.

KEY POINTS

- Nephrotoxicity is commonly caused by drugs whose elimination is dependent on renal function.
- Common risk factors for the development of nephrotoxicity include:
  - Advanced age of the patient
  - Presence of volume depletion
  - Underlying renal insufficiency
  - Prolonged duration of drug therapy
  - Administration of more than one nephrotoxic agent

Protease Inhibitor–Induced Nephrotoxicity

Patients with HIV infection develop ARF for the same reasons as patients without HIV infection. Protease inhibitors have recently been associated with development of ARF. An acute reversible decrease in renal function may occur shortly after initiating therapy with ritonavir. Indinavir is also associated with the development of ARF. Indinavir is excreted by the kidneys, and indinavir crystals form in the urine, especially if the urine is concentrated or of low volume. The crystals may precipitate in renal tissue and may lead to the development of ARF. In addition, patients treated with indinavir may have symptoms such as dysuria, colic, and back pain, since indinavir kidney stones can be associated with urinary tract obstruction and postrenal azotemia. Abnormalities such as hematuria or crystalluria provide clues to the diagnosis. In many patients, therapy with indinavir can be restarted after volume repletion. Crystalluria and intrarenal obstruction may be the cause of ARF in patients treated with sulfadiazine and acyclovir as well as indinavir.

KEY POINTS

- Acute renal failure due to various causes occurs in patients with HIV infection.
- The protease inhibitors are a newly recognized cause of nephrotoxicity in patients with HIV infection.
- Indinavir may cause acute renal failure by several different mechanisms.

Drug-Induced Acute Interstitial Nephritis

- How does acute interstitial nephritis differ from nephrotoxic renal disease?

Although infections and immunologic diseases may cause acute interstitial nephritis, this disorder is most frequently associated with medications. Penicillins, quinolones, nonsteroidal anti-inflammatory drugs, diuretics, cimetidine, phenytoin, phenobarbital, allopurinol, cephalosporins, interferon-alfa, and other drugs have been implicated in the development of acute interstitial nephritis. The diagnosis is suggested by the presence of nonoliguric ARF, especially in association with signs of systemic hypersensitivity, such as fever, rash, and eosinophilia. Sterile pyuria and microscopic hematuria are common findings, and non-nephrotic-range proteinuria may be present. Eosinophiluria is a supportive finding and often differentiates acute interstitial nephritis from acute tubular necrosis, nephrotoxicity, and pyelonephritis. The presence of eosinophils in the urine should be evaluated with either Wright's stain or the more specific Hansel's stain, although eosinophiluria is a nonspecific finding. Eosinophiluria may also occur in patients with acute prostatitis, rapidly progressive glomerulonephritis, and cholesterol emboli. Renal histologic specimens demonstrate an acute interstitial infiltrate composed of mononuclear cells and less often of eosinophils.

Therapy involves discontinuation of the causative agent or treatment of the underlying disease. Although glucocorticoids are often used in the treatment of acute interstitial nephritis, there are no data from prospective clinical trials evaluating the efficacy of this therapy. Recovery is variable in time, and dialysis may be necessary.

KEY POINT

- **Acute interstitial nephritis is an inflammatory disease with characteristic systemic and laboratory findings.**

Acute Renal Failure in Patients with Malignancy

- What causes acute renal failure in patients with malignancy?
- What are the major nephrotoxic drugs given to patients who are being treated for malignancy?
- What are the most common risk factors for the development of ARF in patients with malignancy?
- What therapeutic strategies may be used to limit the development of nephrotoxicity in patients with malignancy?

Urinary tract obstruction should always be considered in patients with malignancy, especially those with lymphoma or pelvic organ neoplasms. Acute oliguric urate nephropathy, a consequence of intratubular deposition of urate crystals, occurs most often in patients with lymphoproliferative and hematologic disorders. Uric acid is soluble at an alkaline urine pH, but its solubility diminishes markedly with a pH of less than 6.5. Hyperuricemia secondary to rapid cell turnover occurs spontaneously in patients with tumor cell lysis or is enhanced after radiation therapy or chemotherapy. ARF due to tumor cell lysis is accompanied by the release of other ions from neoplastic cells, resulting in hyperphosphatemia, hypocalcemia, and hyperkalemia. Uric acid crystalluria and a high urine uric acid:urine creatinine ratio (> 1.0) are found. Preventive therapy includes administering allopurinol before beginning chemotherapy, ensuring volume repletion, and alkalinizing the urine with sodium bicarbonate in an attempt to maintain urine pH above 6.5. Treatment of ARF and other metabolic derangements is associated with a good prognosis.

ARF is common in patients who have undergone bone marrow transplantation. More than 50% of these patients require treatment with dialysis. The use of nephrotoxic chemotherapy and immunosuppressive agents may exacerbate the renal disease. Causes of ARF in bone marrow transplant recipients include prerenal azotemia, tumor cell lysis, nephrotoxicity from bone marrow infusion, sepsis, and administration of amphotericin B. In addition, a hepatorenal-like syndrome, associated with hepatic veno-occlusive disease, may occur 10 to 16 days after bone marrow transplantation. The hepatic disease may be the result of endothelial cell injury caused by radiation therapy and chemotherapeutic agents. Such patients have a urinary sodium concentration of less than 20 to 40 meq/L, which is frequently associated with volume overload. Patients with preexisting liver and renal disease are at high risk for developing this disorder.

The hemolytic–uremic syndrome may occur following bone marrow transplantation. Its clinical presentation is often that of the nephritic syndrome (hypertension, renal insufficiency, proteinuria, and hematuria, often with erythrocyte casts) that occurs 4 to 12 months after bone marrow transplantation. The diagnosis should be suspected in a patient who has microangiopathic hemolytic anemia, thrombocytopenia, and central nervous system dysfunction. Therapy is supportive, and some patients develop end-stage renal disease.

The clinical syndrome of radiation nephropathy includes hypertension, renal insufficiency, renal vascular damage, proteinuria, and anemia. The syndrome develops in patients who received radiation exposure to the kidneys of greater than 23 Gy and often occurs months after completion of the radiation therapy.

Cisplatin (formerly called *cis*-platinum) nephrotoxicity may present as polyuria without azotemia during the first 2 days after drug administration. Nephrogenic diabetes insipidus and a decreased GFR may occur 72 to 96 hours after administration of cisplatin. Recovery usually occurs within 2 to 4 weeks, but renal abnormalities may persist. Cisplatin, nephrotoxicity is dose-dependent and cumulative. Maintaining volume repletion and administering intravenous fluids before and during therapy, limiting the dose of cisplatin, and using diuretics such as furosemide and mannitol to maintain a high urine output may help prevent nephrotoxicity.

Methotrexate causes both acute tubular necrosis and renal failure because of crystal precipitation within renal tubules. Antineoplastic antibiotics such as plicamycin may also cause acute tubular necrosis. Dose-related mitomycin-C toxicity is usually associated with the hemolytic–uremic syndrome.

Biologic response modifiers are increasingly used in the treatment of various neoplastic diseases. Interleukin-2 causes a capillary leak–like syndrome, associated with edema, ascites, and oliguria. Patients have a low FE_{Na}, consistent with prerenal azotemia. Clinical toxicities due to interleukin-2 are dose related and are generally reversible. Renal function usually returns to normal within 30 days after cessation of therapy. Administration of interferon-alfa is rarely associated with the development of non-nephrotic-range proteinuria, but urinary protein levels may reach the nephrotic range. ARF has occurred in a few patients who received interferon-alfa, and interstitial nephritis, minimal change nephropathy, and immune complex nephropathy have all been reported in patients taking this drug. Interferon-gamma has caused ARF (focal segmental glomerulosclerosis and acute tubular necrosis) and proteinuria. Immunoglobulin therapy has been associated with a spectrum of renal disorders including ARF, but the abnormalities are usually reversible. Renal biopsy specimens may show proximal tubular cell injury. Advanced age, volume depletion, and renal insufficiency are risk factors for this complication.

In addition to drugs given to treat opportunistic infections in immunocompromised hosts, immunosuppressive medications such as tacrolimus and cyclosporine can result in the development of renal insufficiency. ARF occurs frequently, is usually dose dependent, and is manifested by vasoconstriction, which is generally reversible if the dose is decreased or the drug is discontinued. Rarely, these drugs may cause a thrombotic microangiopathic ARF.

KEY POINTS

- Urinary tract obstruction should always be considered in patients with malignancy.
- Urinary tract obstruction is associated with lymphoma, gastrointestinal neoplasms, and tumors of the genitourinary system.
- Urate nephropathy may often be prevented in patients who are undergoing chemotherapy by pretreatment with allopurinol.
- Nephropathy following bone marrow transplantation comprises several syndromes.
- Nephropathy may occur shortly or some months after bone marrow transplantation.

Other Causes of Acute Renal Failure

Liver Disease

Patients with liver disease are at risk for developing several types of ARF. The most common cause is prerenal azotemia in patients with cirrhosis and ascites. Patients with liver disease may also develop acute tubular necrosis during periods of hemodynamic instability or sepsis, because of use of nephrotoxins, or secondary to rhabdomyolysis. The hepatorenal syndrome (HRS) is a form of progressive decreased renal perfusion that occurs in patients with advanced liver disease in whom there are no other causes sufficient to explain the severity and persistence of the renal dysfunction (such as drug toxicity, infection, or other underlying systemic illness). HRS is thought to be a physiologic renal response to systemic complications of the liver disease. The mortality rate for patients with HRS is extremely high. Spontaneous recovery occurs rarely, typically if the hepatic disease improves. The severity of the liver disease is probably the most important determinant of survival. Liver transplantation may successfully reverse HRS in this high-risk population.

Although HRS usually occurs in patients with cirrhosis, it may develop in patients with fulminant hepatitis or hepatic malignancy. Patients usually have ascites, portal hypertension, jaundice, hypoalbuminemia, and some degree of hypotension. HRS frequently occurs in conjunction with diuresis, paracentesis, surgical procedures, gastrointestinal bleeding, and infection. To diagnose HRS, volume status must be adequate; volume status is usually measured by central venous pressure and/or cardiac hemodynamic parameters. The urinary sodium concentration is usually less than 10 meq/L, and the FE_{Na} is generally less than 1%. The finding of a high urinary sodium concentration in the absence of diuretic administration strongly suggests another diagnosis. Azotemia and oliguria are progressive. The pathogenesis of HRS is unknown, but abnormalities of leukotriene and endothelin metabolism, shunting of renal plasma flow from cortical to medullary segments, and intense renal vasoconstriction in the presence of systemic vasodilatation have all been implicated. Renal histologic findings do not suggest any structural renal disease as a cause for HRS.

Treatment consists of identifying and discontinuing possible inciting agents and maintaining central and renal hemodynamic parameters, often using albumin infusions to enhance oncotic pressure. Vasodilator or vasopressor agents, such as dopamine or vasopressin, have not proved to be effective. Insertion of peritoneovenous shunts has been advocated for treating HRS, but conclusions from uncontrolled clinical trials may not be valid. Complications of shunts include infection, disseminated intravascular coagulation, and peritoneal leakage. Peritoneovenous shunting is associated with some improvement in renal function, but patient survival is not meaningfully enhanced. Infusion of prostaglandins, dopamine, or ornipressin (a vasopressin analog) does not improve outcome.

Rhabdomyolysis

ARF due to rhabdomyolysis is associated with high serum creatine kinase and creatinine levels, hyperuricemia, hyperkalemia, and hyperphosphatemia. This form of ARF may be precipitated by muscle trauma, strenuous exercise, influenza, potassium or phosphorus depletion, drug overdose, and alcoholism. Drugs such as 3-hydroxy-3-methylglutaryl–coenzyme A (HMG-CoA) inhibitors may also cause ARF due to rhabdomyolysis, especially in patients with inborn errors of muscle metabolism. Recent reports of ARF associated with rhabdomyolysis after cocaine use have described associated hepatic failure and disseminated intravascular coagulation. The serum creatinine level may be markedly increased or rise by more than 2 mg/dL per day as a result of muscle injury and decreased renal excretion. Urinalysis shows dipstick-positive heme in the absence of erythrocytes on microscopic examination, reflecting myoglobinuria. Pigmented casts are also seen. Other microscopic findings are the same as those of acute tubular necrosis.

Volume repletion, administration of mannitol, and administration of sodium bicarbonate to alkalinize the urine have been recommended despite lack of studies showing that these therapeutic measures are effective after the onset of renal injury. Administration of furosemide early in the course of ARF has been suggested for patients with oliguria. The ultimate prognosis is good, although dialysis may be necessary, especially if severe hyperkalemia is present.

Atherosclerotic Heart Disease and Peripheral Vascular Disease

Patients with atherosclerotic heart disease and peripheral vascular disease may be at risk for several types of renal disease. The most common type is prerenal azotemia in patients with congestive heart failure. However, patients with heart disease may develop acute tubular necrosis during periods of hemodynamic instability or sepsis, after receiving nephrotoxic drugs, or following administration of contrast agents during coronary angiography or peripheral arteriography. Atheroembolic renal disease occurs in patients with atherosclerosis, especially after angiography, angioplasty, vascular surgery, treatment with intra-aortic balloon pumps, anticoagulation, or thrombolysis. Renal atheroemboli rarely occur spontaneously. The clinical findings are a result of cholesterol crystals or debris from atheromatous plaques obstructing small renal vessels and causing local inflammation, ischemia, hypertension, and progressive renal insufficiency. Other organ system dysfunction, such as cerebral ischemia, ocular abnormalities, and intestinal vascular insufficiency, may occur concomitantly and are clues to the diagnosis. Refractile plaques in retinal arteries (Hollenhorst plaques), livedo reticularis, petechial lesions, and cyanosis of the lower extremity digits may be noted. Leukocytosis, eosinophilia, eosinophiluria, hypocomplementemia, and an increased erythrocyte sedimentation rate are variable findings and are not diagnostic. The diagnosis may be confirmed by biopsy of muscle, skin, or kidney that shows the typical biconcave clefts left in small vessels.

The course of renal insufficiency varies but is frequently progressive over days to months. No treatment has been shown to be beneficial. Therapy consists of treating hypertension, discontinuing anticoagulation, and preparing for dialysis if necessary. The prognosis for recovery of renal function and patient survival is poor.

Chronic Renal Insufficiency

The progressive loss of renal function may be broadly classified into three categories: chronic renal insufficiency (glomerular filtration rate [GFR] 50 to 25 mL/min), chronic renal failure (GFR 25 to 10 mL/min), and end-stage renal disease (GFR < 10 mL/min) (see Figure 1 in the section on Clinical Evaluation of Renal Function). Table 24 lists the major causes of renal diseases that progress to end-stage renal disease (ESRD). Despite various causes for the original disease, there appears to be a final common pathway for the progression of renal disease and its concomitant metabolic perturbations.

The prevalence of ESRD has increased markedly since the inception of dialysis more than three decades ago. Currently, nearly 300,000 patients are in an ESRD treatment program in the United States (average growth 8% to 9% per

TABLE 24 Causes of End-Stage Renal Disease

Cause	%
Diabetes mellitus	40%
Hypertension	27%
Chronic glomerulonephritis	13%
Renal cystic kidney disease/autosomal dominant polycystic kidney disease	3% to 4%
Interstitial nephritis	4%
Other	12%
Obstructive uropathy	
Lupus nephritis	
HIV	

year) at a cost of more than 15 billion dollars in 1998, with the greatest growth being in the elderly population. A disproportionately high number of minority races are represented; the incidence in black Americans, Mexicans, and native Americans is three to four times that of white Americans. Potential causes for this unequal burden of ESRD include a higher prevalence of diabetes mellitus and hypertension in these minority populations and the possibility of greater genetic susceptibility to renal injury from these causes.

Management Issues in Patients with Chronic Renal Disease

- When is the appropriate time to refer a patient with chronic renal disease to a nephrology consultant?
- What interventions may slow the progression of chronic renal disease?
- Should recombinant erythropoietin be given to patients with chronic renal failure and concomitant anemia?
- What is the optimal therapy for patients with secondary hyperparathyroidism and potential renal bone disease?

Case 17

A 35-year-old man selects you as his new primary care physician. He complains of fatigue. The patient has had type 1 diabetes mellitus since age 8. He also has a 3-year history of hypertension and "a kidney problem." Medications include insulin, enalapril, and ibuprofen as needed.

Physical examination discloses a blood pressure of 148/92 mm Hg (supine and standing), diabetic retinopathy, peripheral sensory neuropathy, and trace pedal edema. Hematocrit is 28%. Plasma glucose is 158 mg/dL. Serum creatinine is 3.3 mg/dL, sodium 136 meq/L, potassium 5.0 meq/L, chloride 100 meq/L, and bicarbonate 20 meq/L. Hemoglobin A_{1c} is 8%. Serum albumin is 3.8 g/dL, calcium 8.2 mg/dL, and phosphorus 5.6 mg/dL. Urinalysis shows 4+ protein without glucose or heme; microscopic examination discloses oval fat bodies. A 24-hour urine specimen shows excretion of protein of 4.8 g/24 h and creatinine clearance of 24 mL/min.

The findings in this case highlight important contemporary management issues in caring for the patient with chronic renal failure. These issues include when to refer to a nephrology consultant, progression of renal disease, management of anemia, treatment of hypertension, role of calcium and phosphorus metabolism, and planning for appropriate care of the patient with ESRD.

Referral to a Nephrology Consultant

A recent National Institutes of Health (NIH) conference emphasized the importance of early referral in an attempt to reduce the substantial morbidity and mortality of patients with renal disease. Conference participants recommended that females with a serum creatinine concentration greater than 1.5 mg/dL and males with a serum creatinine concentration greater than 2.0 mg/dL be referred for nephrology consultation to confirm the diagnosis of renal disease and to initiate appropriate medical therapy for concomitant disorders.

Progression of Renal Disease

In any patient with chronic renal disease, the initial efforts should be directed toward establishing the correct renal diagnosis and identifying any potential reversible factors that may be superimposed on the chronic condition. Such adverse factors are summarized in Table 25. In the patient in Case 17, the clinical presentation is consistent with diabetic nephropathy, and the patient's ibuprofen and any other nonsteroidal anti-inflammatory drugs were discontinued.

TABLE 25 Potentially Reversible Causes of Worsening Renal Failure

Hypotension/renal hypoperfusion
Volume depletion
Congestive heart failure
Nephrotoxic drugs or radiocontrast agents
Urinary tract obstruction
Hypercalcemia
Sepsis
Uncontrolled hypertension

Pathophysiology

In many renal diseases, chronic renal insufficiency may progress even if the initial insult has resolved. For most patients with renal disease, the decline in the GFR is usually linear and can be depicted by serially plotting the reciprocal of the serum creatinine value versus time. Since various renal diseases may result in ESRD, progressive chronic renal insufficiency may be due to secondary factors unrelated to the original disease. Several events are thought to contribute to the progression of renal disease, including focal glomerulosclerosis and interstitial fibrosis; hyperlipidemia; precipitation of calcium phosphate salts in the renal interstitium; enhanced production of cytokines, such as transforming growth factor-beta (TGF-β) and platelet-derived growth factor (PDGF); and stimulation of the renin-angiotensin system.

Hypertension

Controlling systemic hypertension is the most important intervention to slow the progression of established diabetic nephropathy (Peterson et al.). Adherence to a renal diet (such as protein restriction) is less effective (Klahr et al.). In a patient with diabetes mellitus, optimal glycemic control will reduce the initial development of microalbuminuria or overt nephropathy (see Endocrinology Syllabus).

Hypertension usually accompanies progressive renal insufficiency. Systemic hypertension may exacerbate the increased glomerular capillary pressure, leading to progressive glomerulosclerosis. Both animal and human studies have demonstrated that lowering blood pressure and protein excretion retards the progression of chronic renal insufficiency. Angiotensin-converting enzyme (ACE) inhibitors have been particularly effective in slowing progression of renal insufficiency in patients with and without diabetes mellitus by reducing angiotensin II effects on renal hemodynamics, local growth factors, and perhaps glomerular permselectivity (Giatras et al.; Maschio et al.). Nondihydropyridine calcium channel blockers have also been shown to retard progression of renal insufficiency in patients with type 2 diabetes mellitus.

Target blood pressure should be < 130/85 mm Hg for all patients with renal disease, and a target blood pressure of < 125/75 mm Hg is recommended for patients with proteinuric renal disease (urinary protein ≥ 1 g/24 h). The

Peterson JC, Adler S, Burkart JM, Greene T, Hebert LA, Hunsicker LG, et al. Blood pressure control, proteinuria, and the progression of renal disease. The modification of diet in renal disease study. Ann Intern Med. 1995;123:754-62. UI: 96030745

Klahr S, Levey AS, Beck GJ, Caggiula AW, Hunsicker L, Kusek JW, et al. The effects of dietary protein restriction and blood-pressure control on the progression of chronic renal disease. Modification of Diet in Renal Disease Study Group. N Engl J Med. 1994;330:877-84. UI: 94159010

Giatras I, Lau J, Levey AS. Effect of angiotensin-converting enzyme inhibitors on the progression of nondiabetic renal disease: a meta-analysis of randomized trials. Angiotensin-Converting-Enzyme Inhibition and Progressive Renal Disease Study Group. Ann Intern Med. 1997;127:337-45. UI: 97410747

Maschio G, Alberti D, Janin G, Locatelli F, Mann JF, Motolese M, et al. Effect of the angiotensin-converting-enzyme inhibitor benazepril on the progression of chronic renal insufficiency. The Angiotensin-Converting-Enzyme Inhibition in Progressive Renal Insufficiency Study Group. N Engl J Med. 1996;334:939-45. UI: 96175229 benefit of aggressive blood pressure control is most pronounced in patients with a urinary protein concentration of > 3 g/24 h and benefits patients with both diabetic and nondiabetic renal disease. In patients with type 1 diabetic nephropathy, ACE inhibitors have been demonstrated to have greater renoprotective effects than other antihypertensive agents. Therapy for the patient in Case 17 should include salt restriction, an ACE inhibitor, and a loop diuretic. The role of angiotensin II receptor blockers as an alternative to ACE inhibitors is under study. A calcium channel blocker (preferentially diltiazem or verapamil) may provide additional antihypertensive benefit and may be a reasonable substitute when an ACE inhibitor cannot be used.

Dietary Protein Restriction

The benefit of dietary protein restriction in patients with chronic renal failure remains controversial (Kasiske et al.; Martinez-Maldonado and Sattin; Pedrini et al.). Restricting dietary protein to 0.6 to 1 g/kg/day appears to be safe because it is well tolerated and does not lead to malnutrition unless the patient has severe nephrotic syndrome or chronic advanced renal failure. However, the favorable effect of protein restriction noted in early experimental studies using animal models and patients with diabetes mellitus could not be proved in two large controlled clinical trials of patients without diabetes in Italy and the United States. Nevertheless, a reasonable management recommendation would include rigorous blood pressure control and moderate protein intake. As chronic renal failure progresses, the typical renal diet should also contain 2 g of potassium and 2 g of sodium daily plus the usual fluid intake, especially for patients with hyperkalemia.

Kasiske BL, Lakatua JD, Ma JZ, Louis TA. A meta-analysis of the effects of dietary protein restriction on the rate of decline in renal function. Am J Kidney Dis. 1998;31:954-61. UI: 98293600

Martinez-Maldonado M, Sattin RW. Rate of progression of renal disease and low-protein diet. Am J Kidney Dis. 1998;31:1048-9. UI: 98293614

Pedrini MT, Levey AS, Lau J, Chalmers TC, Wang PH. The effect of dietary protein restriction on the progression of diabetic and nondiabetic renal diseases: a meta-analysis. Ann Intern Med. 1996;124:627-32. UI: 96201235

Anemia

Anemia often accompanies progressive renal insufficiency and is usually due to a deficiency of erythropoietin. The interstitial cells of the normal kidney are the primary sites of erythropoietin synthesis in response to decreased renal tissue oxygenation. The normocytic, normochromic anemia of chronic renal failure is attributable to reduced erythropoietin production as a result of a reduction in functioning renal mass. Other causes of anemia, such as gastrointestinal bleeding, iron or folate deficiency, and hemolysis, may also occur in patients with chronic renal insufficiency.

In patients with ESRD and pre-ESRD, use of recombinant erythropoietin therapy has nearly eliminated anemia as a major cause of morbidity. The response to therapy may be limited by inadequate iron stores, bone marrow fibrosis, or chronic inflammation. Achieving a target hematocrit value of 33% to 36% may improve quality of life and induce regression of left ventricular hypertrophy. Reduction in mortality remains to be demonstrated in a large randomized clinical trial. Potential side effects of erythropoietin therapy include worsening hypertension (approximately 30% of patients), headaches (15%), and a flu-like syndrome (5%).

Patients with chronic renal failure and a hematocrit value of < 30% are candidates for recombinant erythropoietin therapy once a diagnosis of iron deficiency has been excluded. Therefore, the patient in Case 17 would qualify for therapy. However, studies evaluating the putative benefit of recombinant erythropoietin on morbidity and mortality are not available. For patients with severe anemia or anemia-dependent angina, a total erythropoietin dose of 5000 to 10,000 units subcutaneously weekly in divided doses appears warranted. Recombinant erythropoietin has not been shown to have any adverse effects in patients with progressive chronic renal insufficiency due to systemic or intraglomerular capillary hypertension as long as blood pressure is adequately controlled (NFK-DOQI clinical practice guidelines).

Hyperparathyroidism and Renal Osteodystrophy

The development of secondary hyperparathyroidism with resultant renal osteodystrophy is almost universal in patients with chronic renal failure. Phosphate retention begins to occur when the GFR falls. Retention of phosphate plays a central role in stimulating the increase in parathyroid hormone (PTH) synthesis. It is thought to promote PTH release by: 1) the effect of hypocalcemia, 2) the decreased formation and effect of calcitriol [1,25-dihydroxyvitamin D], or 3) the direct effect of hyperphosphatemia on *PTH* gene expression. The effect of hypocalcemia may be sensed directly by the parathyroid gland, as a calcium-sensing receptor with its attendant mRNA and protein has recently been identified. The suppression of renal calcitriol synthesis may increase PTH by lowering the serum calcium concentration and/or by removing the inhibitory effect of calcitriol on the parathyroid gland. Independent of the mechanism, this secondary hyperparathyroid response is a "trade-off" to normalize serum calcium, phosphorus, and calcitriol concentrations at the expense of a persistently elevated PTH concentration and potential bone disease.

Initial therapy should include dietary phosphorus restriction and oral calcium-containing phosphate binders (calcium acetate or calcium carbonate taken with meals) to normalize serum calcium and phosphorus levels. Calcitriol supplements should be used in patients with persistent hypocalcemia or severe hyperparathyroidism. Calcitriol administration has been shown to suppress PTH secretion and to decrease the development of osteomalacia in patients with chronic renal failure. The goal of therapy is to maintain PTH levels at two to three times normal to overcome skeletal resistance to PTH, while avoiding excessive hyperparathyroidism. Intact PTH (or *N*-terminal PTH) should be measured, rather than the inactive *C*-terminal PTH, which accumulates in patients with renal failure.

There are three types of renal bone disease: 1) *osteitis fibrosa* with increased bone turnover due to secondary hyperparathyroidism, 2) *osteomalacia* with low bone turnover and increased osteoid formation secondary to aluminum deposition in bone, and 3) the more recently described *adynamic bone disease*, which may be more prevalent in elderly patients, patients with diabetes mellitus being treated with aluminum hydroxide, and patients on continuous ambulatory peritoneal dialysis (Hruska and Teitelbaum). The pathophysiology of adynamic bone disease may relate to excessive suppression of PTH by calcitriol therapy. Patients with renal osteodystrophy may present with bone pain or fractures. Radiographic signs of osteitis fibrosa include subperiosteal bone resorption of phalanges, distal clavicles, and skull. Osteopenia and pseudofractures are more suggestive of osteomalacia (see Endocrine Syllabus).

Medical Management of the Uremic State

Despite optimal management of chronic renal failure, renal disease eventually progresses and metabolic complications increase. Hypertension and edema due to retention of sodium and water are common and require dietary sodium restriction and diuretics. Since hyperkalemia becomes more likely when the GFR is < 20 mL/min, dietary potassium should be restricted and salt substitutes that might cause hyperkalemia should be avoided. Similarly, magnesium ingestion (particularly magnesium-containing antacids and cathartics) should be restricted. All drugs should be reviewed to see if dose reduction is needed to prevent excessive accumulation. Dosages should be modified consistent with

NKF-DOQI clinical practice guidelines for hemodialysis adequacy. National Kidney Foundation. Am J Kidney Dis. 1997; 30:S15-66. UI: 97438770

KEY POINTS

- **Early referral to a nephrologist for patients with azotemia (serum creatinine level > 2.0 mg/dL for males and 1.5 mg/dL for females) is recommended in an attempt to reduce the substantial morbidity and mortality of patients with renal disease.**
- **Adequate control of systemic hypertension is the most important intervention to slow the progression of renal insufficiency. Target blood pressure should be < 130/85 mm Hg in all patients with renal disease and < 125/75 mm Hg in patients with urinary protein concentration > 1 g/24 h. ACE inhibitors appear to have a renoprotective effect.**
- **Therapy with erythropoietin is effective in correcting the anemia of chronic renal disease in patients with pre–end-stage renal disease and end-stage renal disease.**
- **The three types of renal bone disease are 1) osteitis fibrosa with increased bone turnover due to secondary hyperparathyroidism, 2) osteomalacia with low bone turnover and increased osteoid formation secondary to aluminum deposition in bone, and 3) adynamic bone disease.**
- **Management strategies to prevent renal osteodystrophy include 1) dietary phosphorus restriction, 2) oral calcium-containing phosphorus binders, and 3) calcitriol supplements to increase serum calcium and suppress parathyroid hormone secretion.**

Hruska KA, Teitelbaum SL. Renal osteodystrophy. N Engl J Med. 1995;333:166-74. UI: 95312014 excretion of the drugs by the failing kidneys. Correction of metabolic acidosis may lessen the adverse effects of secondary hyperparathyroidism on bone.

Uremia is the term reserved for clinical signs and symptoms related to advanced azotemia and includes fatigue, sleep disturbances, loss of appetite, nausea, vomiting, pruritus, pericarditis, neuropathy, the restless legs syndrome, asterixis, and seizures. Uremia does not usually appear until the GFR has decreased to < 10 mL/min but may appear earlier in patients with diabetes mellitus.

Uremia results in several endocrine abnormalities, including resistance to insulin and growth hormone, impaired production of 1,25-dihydroxyvitamin D and testosterone, hyperprolactinemia, and altered thyroxine metabolism. Renal insulin clearance is decreased, which allows many patients with diabetes mellitus to reduce their insulin dose or discontinue insulin entirely. As a result of these abnormalities, infertility, amenorrhea, and sexual dysfunction are common in adults with ESRD, and growth retardation frequently occurs in children with ESRD.

Peripheral neuropathy can occur in patients with uremia. Initiation of dialysis may halt the progression of the neuropathy, but dialysis will not be as successful as renal transplantation in correcting this disorder. In patients with diabetes mellitus, signs of autonomic neuropathy (especially gastroparesis) increase as renal insufficiency progresses. Uremic seizures and coma are indications for immediate dialysis.

Table 26 lists absolute and relative indications and contraindications for initiating renal replacement therapy.

Treatment Options for Patients with End-Stage Renal Disease

- What are the merits of renal transplantation versus dialysis in patients with end-stage renal disease?

Once ESRD develops, patient choices include dialysis (peritoneal or hemodialysis), renal transplantation, or death without treatment. The importance of early referral to a nephrologist cannot be overemphasized. Early referral allows ample time for patient education and preparation for various treatment options and provides a smooth transition to therapy. The patient's primary internist may play a pivotal role in initiating this process and may also help counsel patients with terminal or severely debilitating disease who may wish to decline dialysis.

TABLE 26 Indications and Contraindications for Renal Replacement Therapy in End-Stage Renal Disease
Absolute Indications
Hyperkalemia
Congestive heart failure
Refractory metabolic acidosis
Pericarditis
Relative Indications
Glomerular filtration rate ≤ 10 mL/min (or ≤ 15 mL/min in a patient with diabetes mellitus)
Serum creatinine ≥ 8 mg/dL (or ≥ 6 mg/dL in a patient with diabetes mellitus)
Uremic symptoms
Relative Contraindications
Severe irreversible dementia
Debilitating chronic disease

Dialysis versus Renal Transplantation

Patients should be counseled about their options for dialysis or transplantation and receive information comparing survival and quality of life with both modalities. For dialysis patients, the overall mortality rates approximate 22% at 1 year and 60% to 70% at 5 years for patients without diabetes mellitus. Mortality rates are greater for diabetic patients. Recent data comparing survival of patients matched for age and renal disease have shown a clear survival advantage for cadaveric renal transplantation compared with dialysis. There is also ample evidence documenting a superior quality of life after transplantation. Unfortunately, not all patients are well enough to qualify for transplantation. The current shortage of donor organs in the United States severely limits patient access to cadaveric transplantation despite the superior results and reduced long-term costs associated with this modality. At the end of 1998, more than 41,000 patients were on the cadaveric renal transplantation waiting list. To avoid prolonged waiting, patients are now encouraged to find their own donor because excellent results are achieved with kidneys from both living related and unrelated donors (including a patient's spouse).

Dialysis

Dialysis treatment options include home hemodialysis, in-center hemodialysis, and home peritoneal dialysis (either chronic ambulatory or cycler peritoneal dialysis). In the United States, in-center hemodialysis is used for nearly 85% of patients, peritoneal dialysis for 15%, and home hemodialysis for only 1%. There is no significant difference in survival when either chronic ambulatory peritoneal dialysis or in-center hemodialysis is used for patients who do not have diabetes mellitus. A recent report suggests an increase in mortality when chronic ambulatory peritoneal dialysis is used for diabetic patients and the elderly.

Patient choice regarding the type of dialysis may depend on several factors. Patients who want to assume maximum control over their own care should choose home dialysis – usually peritoneal dialysis. Access for peritoneal dialysis requires the placement of a peritoneal catheter 2 to 4 weeks before starting therapy. Peritonitis (usually caused by gram-positive organisms) is the major risk of this modality, although the frequency of peritonitis has been reduced to one episode per 18-patient-months because of improved aseptic techniques. Hemodialysis requires the creation of an arteriovenous fistula or a prosthetic vascular graft weeks to months prior to initiation of dialysis (Ifudu). Despite its greater longevity and fewer complications of thrombosis and infection, the use of a native arteriovenous fistula has declined. A central catheter, preferably placed in the internal jugular vein, may also be used for acute hemodialysis; however, infection and thrombosis are more common.

Ifudu O. Current concepts: Care of patients undergoing hemodialysis. N Engl J Med. 1998;339:1054-62. UI: 98425651

Medical Problems in Dialysis Patients

Anemia, bone disease, and hypertension persist despite dialysis and require continued attention. Exogenous erythropoietin and calcitriol are administered intravenously during dialysis treatment. Cardiovascular disease and infection (sepsis, pneumonia, access site infection) are the leading causes of morbidity and mortality. Ischemic heart disease, cardiomyopathy, and left ventricular hypertrophy due to hypertension frequently occur in patients undergoing dialysis, and anemia is a common finding. Cardiovascular risk factors include the presence of hypertension, diabetes mellitus, hyperlipidemia, hyperhomocystinemia, and reduced lipoprotein(a) concentration. When definitive treatment of coronary obstruction is required, coronary artery bypass surgery is preferred because restenosis rates of up to 70% to 80% at 6 months have been reported following coronary angioplasty in patients undergoing dialysis.

Patients in the United States who are undergoing dialysis have inferior survival rates compared with patients in several other countries. Possible explanations include poor patient selection, adverse psychosocial characteristics, and an inadequate amount of time spent undergoing dialysis. Close monitoring of the intensity and duration of dialysis is now done routinely for each patient, and delivery of the dialysate is maintained at a dose thought to be associated with improved survival. Increasing the dose of dialysate is usually accomplished by increasing the amount of time on hemodialysis or by increasing the volume exchanged for patients receiving peritoneal dialysis.

Renal Transplantation

Transplantation is considered successful when a GFR of > 50 mL/min is achieved. In addition to improved survival, the benefits of successful transplantation include resolution of anemia; return of normal endocrine, sexual, and reproductive function; and enhancement of energy levels, making return to full-time employment and more strenuous physical activity feasible. In diabetic patients, autonomic neuropathy with gastroparesis, gastroenteropathy, and postural hypotension persist or worsen on dialysis, yet stabilize or improve after renal transplantation. Major disadvantages of renal transplantation include the surgical risk and side effects and the cost of immunosuppressants.

Contraindications to Renal Transplantation

There is currently no absolute age limit prohibiting renal transplantation, although older patients are more likely to have a medical problem that would exclude them from receiving a transplant. The most frequently used exclusion criteria are summarized in Table 27. In addition, patients who are substance abusers or are noncompliant while undergoing dialysis are usually excluded from undergoing renal transplantation until they demonstrate a period of abstinence or improved compliance.

TABLE 27 Exclusion Criteria for Renal Transplantation

Active infection* (including HIV)
Recent malignancy
Dementia
Significant cardiopulmonary or hepatic disease
Chronically debilitated state
Habitual substance abuse or noncompliance

*Hepatitis C is controversial

Patient and Graft Survival

Overall *patient* survivals of 95% at 1 year and 88% at 5 years after transplantation are expected. Survival is highest in young, otherwise healthy patients and lowest in older patients with diabetes mellitus. Major causes of mortality include cardiovascular disease (the leading cause of death), infection, liver disease, and malignancy. Cadaveric *graft* survivals of 85% at 1 year and 70% at 5 years after renal transplantation can now be expected with the use of newer immunosuppressants. Graft survival is better in recipients of living (related and unrelated) kidneys and is reduced in recipients of a second kidney, in highly sensitized patients, and in black Americans. For patients under 45 years of age with type 1 diabetes mellitus but without cardiovascular disease, the 1-year patient and allograft survival rates in recipients of simultaneous kidney/pancreas transplants are comparable to those in recipients of cadaveric kidney allografts alone. Patients with diabetes who are eligible for a living-related kidney allograft would do well to choose pancreas transplantation *after* living-related kidney transplantation, provided they are willing to wait for a well-matched pancreas. Acute rejection continues to be the major reason for loss of the renal allograft within the first 2 years. In addition to the improvement in short-term cadaveric graft survival, long-term survival has also improved (Hariharan et al.).

Hariharan S, Johnson CP, Bresnahan BA, Taranto SE, McIntosh MJ, Stablein D. Improved graft survival after renal transplantation in the United States, 1988 to 1996. N Engl J Med. 2000;342:605-12. UI: 20143074

Special Problems in Renal Transplant Recipients

The early risks and morbidity of renal transplantation are due primarily to acute rejection and to the effects of immunosuppressants used to prevent graft rejection. Although cyclosporine and prednisone (with or without azathioprine) continue to be used in most centers, newer agents are also available. Tacrolimus acts similarly to cyclosporine (inhibiting interleukin-2 production) and has a

Uric Acid Stone Disease

Uric acid stones occur predominantly in patients with unusually low urine pH and hyperuricosuria. In some patients, this abnormal urine pH is due to a defect in renal ammonia secretion, which results in less buffering of secreted hydrogen ion and very low urine pH. Uric acid stones are radiolucent but are visualized by both ultrasonography and CT. Since the solubility of uric acid is greatly increased when urine pH is elevated, treatment should consist of hydration and alkalinization of the urine to pH > 6.5 with oral sodium bicarbonate or sodium citrate solution. When hyperuricosuria is present, a low-purine diet and/or administration of allopurinol is indicated.

Cystine Stone Disease

Cystine stone disease occurs in individuals who have inherited an autosomal recessive gastrointestinal and renal tubular transport disorder of four amino acids — cystine, ornithine, arginine, and lysine. Of these, cystine is the most insoluble in normally acid urine and thus precipitates into stones. Onset occurs at a younger age than the onset of calcium stone disease. Cystine stones are radiopaque. Treatment consists of hydration, alkalinization of the urine to pH 6.5, and administration of D-penicillamine or α-mercaptopropionyl glycine (Thiola) to convert the cystine to a more soluble cysteine–drug disulfide complex. Some studies have shown that captopril has effects similar to those of D-penicillamine.

Workup and Management of Patients with Nephrolithiasis

Most renal stones are composed of calcium, are smaller that 5 mm, and will readily pass without instrumentation. Evaluation of the first stone in an adult should include a family history, routine serum chemistry panel, urinalysis, and intravenous pyelography or renal ultrasonography to look for multiple stones or anatomic abnormalities of the urinary tract. Treatment for a first uncomplicated calcium stone is hydration and observation. However, nephrolithiasis recurs in many patients. Additional stones will form in 35% of patients in 2 years and in 52% of patients in 10 years.

Workup for recurrent or complicated stones includes questioning about use of over-the-counter vitamins, chronic dehydration, diarrheal disorders, sarcoidosis, and conditions associated with renal tubular acidosis (such as Sjögren's syndrome). Diagnostic studies include intravenous pyelography; determination of serum creatinine, calcium, uric acid, and electrolytes (looking for renal tubular acidosis); determination of serum parathyroid hormone and 1,25-dihydroxyvitamin D levels (especially in patients with hypercalcemia); urine culture; and 24-hour urine collection for sodium, calcium oxalate, urate, and citrate. Nephrocalcinosis on radiographs suggests the presence of hyperparathyroidism, medullary sponge kidney, or renal tubular acidosis. Hypercalcemia that develops after treatment with a thiazide diuretic for hypercalciuria suggests the presence of latent hyperparathyroidism. Onset of stone disease in patients under the age of 20 years suggests a diagnosis of cystinuria or renal tubular acidosis. A family history of renal stones is more common in patients with idiopathic hypercalciuria and cystinuria.

Basic treatment regardless of stone type includes high fluid intake, relief of persistent obstruction, and treatment of infection. In patients with idiopathic calcium stone disease, hypercalciuria is managed by dietary sodium restriction (but not calcium restriction), thiazide diuretics, and/or amiloride (Ruml et al.). Hyperoxaluria may respond to dietary oxalate restriction. In patients with cal-

Ruml LA, Pearle MS, Pak CY. Medical therapy: calcium oxalate urolithiasis. Urol Clin North Am. 1997;24:117-33. UI: 97201027

Jaeger P. Prevention of recurrent calcium stones: diet versus drugs. Miner Electrolyte Metab. 1994;20:410-3. UI: 95303066

KEY POINT

- **A workup for recurrent nephrolithiasis should include:**
  - **Medical history: urinary tract infection, diarrhea, gout**
  - **Family history: cystinuria, oxalosis**
  - **Determination of urine pH**
  - **Urine culture, if indicated**
  - **Determination of serum calcium and phosphorus levels**
  - **Determination of serum parathyroid hormone and 1,25-dihydroxyvitamin D levels**
  - **Renal imaging: ultrasonography, intravenous pyelography, spiral CT**
  - **Stone analysis**
  - **24-Hour urine: calcium, sodium, oxalate, citrate, urate, and creatinine**

cium stone disease, treatment of coexisting hyperuricosuria with either a low-purine diet or allopurinol reduces the frequency of recurrent calcium stones (Jaeger). Treatment of isolated idiopathic hypocitraturia with oral citrate is not of proven benefit.

Renal Function and Disease in Pregnancy

- What is the significance of electrolyte abnormalities and increased urinary protein excretion in pregnant women?
- What is the significance of and clinical approach to asymptomatic bacteriuria in pregnant women?

In normal pregnancy, blood pressure falls soon after conception and reaches a nadir at about 20 weeks. This drop in blood pressure results from an imbalance between peripheral vasodilatation, which is associated with increased synthesis of vasodilatory prostacyclin (prostaglandin I_2, PGI_2) and vasoconstriction, which is mediated by increased thromboxane synthesis (Chapman et al.). Cardiac output, blood and plasma volume, and sodium retention increase during pregnancy. Edema commonly occurs. Renal size increases and ureteral dilatation develops. Renal plasma flow increases 50% to 70% above normal during the first trimester and remains elevated during the second and third trimesters. The glomerular filtration rate (GFR) increases at the end of the first month of pregnancy, rising to over 150% of normal, and remains elevated until term. These hemodynamic events cause a low-normal blood urea nitrogen level (mean, 7.5 to 10.0 mg/dL) and serum creatinine concentration (mean, 0.5 to 0.8 mg/dL) and a low uric acid level. Therefore, serum creatinine and blood pressure values at the upper limits of normal in nonpregnant patients are abnormal in pregnant women. Urinary protein excretion rarely exceeds 200 mg/24 h, but glucosuria in the absence of hyperglycemia is common.

Asymptomatic bacteriuria develops in approximately 5% of pregnant women. The bacteriuria should be treated, since it may be associated with premature labor and delivery and infants who are small for gestational age. Bacteriuria may progress to pyelonephritis in up to one third of patients. Pyelonephritis is associated with an increased risk of intrauterine death and premature labor. Women with asymptomatic bacteriuria should have regular urine cultures after completion of antibiotic therapy, whereas women with pyelonephritis should receive chronic suppressive antibiotic therapy.

Chapman AB, Abraham WT, Zamudio S, Coffin C, Merouani A, Young D, et al. Temporal relationships between hormonal and hemodynamic changes in early human pregnancy. Kidney Int. 1998;54:2056-63. UI: 99070383

KEY POINTS

- **Blood pressure falls soon after conception.**
- **The glomerular filtration rate increases at the end of the first month of pregnancy and remains elevated until term.**
- **Normal blood urea nitrogen and serum creatinine levels may be associated with significant renal dysfunction in pregnant patients.**
- **Urinary protein excretion rarely exceeds 200 mg/24 h during pregnancy.**
- **Asymptomatic bacteriuria is common in pregnant patients and should be treated.**

Hypertension During Pregnancy

- What is the differential diagnosis of and the complications associated with hypertension during pregnancy?
- How should hypertension be treated during pregnancy?

Hypertension during pregnancy is defined as blood pressure of 140/90 mm Hg or greater, or an increase in systolic blood pressure of 30 mm Hg or diastolic blood pressure of 15 mm Hg compared with values before 20 weeks of gestation. Hypertension affects approximately 10% of pregnant women. The differential diagnosis includes preexisting essential or secondary hypertension (which may be masked by the vasodilatation of pregnancy), transient hypertension, preeclampsia, and chronic hypertension with superimposed preeclampsia (Table 29) (Case Records, Massachusetts General Hosp.). Hypertension that was present before pregnancy or that developed before 20 weeks of gestation must be differentiated from hypertension complicating pregnancy after the

Case records of the Massachusetts General Hospital. Weekly clinicopathological exercises. Case 30-1998. A 30-year-old woman with increasing hypertension and proteinuria. N Engl J Med. 1998;339:906-13. UI: 98414376

20th week because of the different prognosis and treatment of preeclampsia. The presence of hypertensive retinopathy and electrocardiographic changes or the absence of nephrotic-range proteinuria may be helpful in confirming a diagnosis of chronic hypertension. This disorder affects from 1% to 5% of pregnant patients and is more common in older, obese, and black women. Blood pressure > 120/75 mm Hg is associated with increased fetal and maternal morbidity and mortality. Preexisting hypertension increases the risk of preeclampsia, abruptio placentae, fetal growth retardation, and fetal death.

Recent studies have identified a mutation in the mineralocorticoid receptor that causes early-onset hypertension that is exacerbated during pregnancy (Geller et al.). The mutation allows progesterone and other circulating steroids to function as receptor agonists. It is unknown how frequently this mutation is a cause of hypertension during pregnancy.

Pregnant patients with chronic hypertension have a 25% to 27% risk of developing preeclampsia, but the frequency of preeclampsia is unrelated to the presence of proteinuria during the first trimester or to subsequent treatment with low-dose aspirin. Women who have a history of preeclampsia, who have had hypertension for at least 4 years prior to pregnancy, or who had a diastolic blood pressure reading of 100 to 110 mm Hg early in pregnancy develop preeclampsia more frequently (Sibai et al.).

Pregnant women with preexisting essential hypertension should be treated, as treatment may improve maternal and fetal outcomes. However, several clinical trials of antihypertensive therapy during pregnancy have not shown a reduced incidence of preeclampsia or premature delivery when hypertensive agents are administered. Bedrest often is effective in lowering diastolic blood pressure to 90 to 100 mm Hg. Sodium restriction is controversial and should only be considered if it was useful during a patient's prior pregnancy. Methyldopa, labetalol, hydralazine, β-blockers, and, more recently, calcium channel blockers have been used to treat women with essential hypertension during pregnancy. Angiotensin-converting enzyme (ACE) inhibitors and angiotensin II receptor blockers should be discontinued because of the occurrence of fetal complications when these medications are taken during the second and third trimesters. The use of diuretics in the treatment of pregnant patients is controversial. Women with chronic hypertension should be monitored frequently after the 20th week for signs of preeclampsia. Transient or "gestational" hypertension develops late in pregnancy, is not associated with signs of preeclampsia, and resolves following delivery. It is more common in multiparous or overweight patients and in women with a family history of hypertension. There are insufficient data from clinical trials to establish precise goals for the level of blood pressure control in such patients.

Some studies have reported that calcium supplementation during pregnancy has beneficial effects on blood pressure and reduces the risk of developing preeclampsia but has no effect on the frequency of preterm or cesarean delivery, intrauterine growth retardation, and intrauterine or perinatal death. Such findings are still controversial.

Preeclampsia and Eclampsia

- What are preeclampsia and eclampsia and how are they diagnosed?
- How is the diagnosis of preeclampsia made in pregnant women with chronic renal disease?
- What are the outcomes and treatment options for patients with preeclampsia or eclampsia?

TABLE 29 Hypertension in Pregnancy
Chronic hypertension (preexisting essential or other types of hypertension)
Preeclampsia and eclampsia
Chronic hypertension with superimposed preeclampsia
Transient hypertension

Reprinted with permission from the National Kidney Foundation. Greenberg A, ed. Primer on Kidney Diseases, 2nd ed. San Diego: Academic Press; 1998. UI:9717616

Geller DS, Farshi A, Pinkerton N, Fradley M, Moritz M, Spitzer A, et al. Activating mineralocorticoid receptor mutation in hypertension exacerbated by pregnancy. Science. 2000;289:119-23. UI: 20342438.

Sibai BM, Lindheimer M, Hauth J, Caritis S, VanDorsten P, Klebanoff M, et al. Risk factors for preeclampsia, abruptio placentae, and adverse neonatal outcomes among women with chronic hypertension. National Institute of Child Health and Human Development Network of Maternal-Fetal Medicine Units. N Engl J Med. 1998;339:667-71. UI: 98383829

KEY POINTS

- **It is important to differentiate hypertension present before pregnancy or developing before 20 weeks of gestation from hypertension complicating pregnancy after the 20th week because of the different prognosis and treatment of preeclampsia.**
- **Physical examination and laboratory studies can provide evidence supporting a diagnosis of chronic hypertension.**
- **Multisystem involvement suggests a diagnosis of preeclampsia.**
- **Preexisting hypertension increases the risk for development of preeclampsia and maternal and infant morbidity.**
- **Hypertension should be treated because maternal and fetal outcomes may be improved as a result of therapy. However, treatment of hypertension in pregnant patients has not reduced the incidence of preeclampsia or premature delivery.**
- **Methyldopa is the drug that has been used the longest for treating hypertension in pregnant patients.**
- **Drugs that interfere with the action of angiotensin should be discontinued in pregnant patients.**

Preeclampsia is a multisystem disease unique to pregnancy. It involves both hypertension and renal disease and is manifested by proteinuria, renal insufficiency, and edema. Preeclampsia is occasionally accompanied by abnormalities of coagulation, but hematuria is unusual. The occurrence of convulsions in patients with preeclampsia defines eclampsia. Preeclampsia usually occurs after the 20th week of gestation, most commonly in women who are pregnant for the first time. When preeclampsia occurs in the first trimester, it strongly suggests that the patient has a hydatidiform mole. The pathogenesis of the disease is unclear, but it may be related to uteroplacental hypoperfusion, an imbalance between increased synthesis of thromboxane and decreased production of prostaglandin I_2 (PGI_2), increased oxidative stress, disordered endothelin metabolism, or endothelial cell dysfunction. The signs and symptoms are the result of widespread effects on endothelial cells.

The diagnosis of preeclampsia is difficult in patients with preexisting renal disease because of the similarity of their signs and symptoms. Reduced urinary creatinine concentrations and uric acid clearance are common and result in elevated serum creatinine and uric acid levels. Weight gain and edema formation may be related to changes in capillary permeability as well as to sodium retention. Serum uric acid levels > 5.5 mg/dL are usually associated with preeclampsia. The level correlates with the severity of clinical and pathologic disease and inversely with fetal survival. Endotheliosis typically develops. This is a renal lesion involving swelling of glomerular endothelial cells, accompanied by glomerular deposition of fibrinogen and infiltration of lipid-laden macrophages. These changes resolve soon after delivery.

Therapy consists of bedrest, antihypertensive agents, seizure prophylaxis as necessary, and, ultimately, delivery. Antihypertensive treatment should be instituted when diastolic blood pressure exceeds 100 mm Hg. Methyldopa, labetalol, and hydralazine have been used, as have calcium channel blockers, β-blockers, and clonidine. Magnesium sulfate, a vasodilator that increases PGI_2 levels, is effective as both a prophylactic agent and an anticonvulsant in patients with preeclampsia. Magnesium sulfate is more effective than phenytoin in preventing seizures in patients with preeclampsia. For unknown reasons, fetal outcome is also better in mothers treated with magnesium sulfate than in mothers treated with other anticonvulsants. Magnesium supplementation has been associated with respiratory paralysis and maternal death. Synergism between magnesium and calcium channel blockers, such as nifedipine, can cause severe hypotension, which should be avoided because of the risk of increasing uteroplacental ischemia. Management of magnesium supplementation may be problematic in pregnant patients with renal disease. Such patients need frequent assessments of neurologic status and serum magnesium concentration. If blood pressure cannot be controlled or if hyperuricemia, proteinuria, or increasing renal insufficiency develops, delivery should be considered even if the fetus is less than 32 weeks old. If eclampsia or the HELLP syndrome (hemolysis, elevated liver enzymes, and thrombocytopenia [low platelets]) develops, immediate delivery is indicated.

In patients at high risk for developing preeclampsia (those with hypertension, diabetes mellitus, preexisting renal disease, multiple pregnancies, poor previous obstetric histories, or family or personal history of preeclampsia), preventive treatment with aspirin, 60 mg daily, may be effective, perhaps by reversing disordered prostaglandin metabolism. Such therapy was reported to decrease the incidence of preeclampsia in healthy women who had never been pregnant before, but was associated with a higher incidence of abruptio placentae. The findings of a benefit associated with aspirin in other populations at risk for the development of preeclampsia, including nulliparous women, have

KEY POINTS

- Therapy for preeclampsia consists of bedrest, antihypertensive agents, seizure prophylaxis, and delivery.
- If fetal maturity is adequate, delivery is the treatment of choice.
- Antihypertensive treatment is instituted when diastolic blood pressure exceeds 100 mm Hg.
- Methyldopa, labetalol, hydralazine, calcium channel blockers, β-blockers, and clonidine have been used to treat hypertension in pregnant women.
- Magnesium sulfate is effective as both a seizure prophylactic and an anticonvulsant.
- It is extremely difficult to diagnose preeclampsia in pregnant patients with preexisting renal disease.
- The development of hyperreflexia or signs of the systemic findings of preeclampsia may be critical clues to the presence of this disorder.
- If blood pressure in patients with preeclampsia cannot be controlled or if hyperuricemia, proteinuria, or increasing renal insufficiency develops, delivery should be considered even if fetal age is less than 32 weeks.

not been confirmed. Such therapy is usually not recommended for patients without risk factors. Administration of the antioxidant vitamins C and E may decrease the incidence of preeclampsia in high-risk patients (Chappell et al.).

The frequency of abruptio placentae and the incidence of preterm delivery, neonatal complications (including rate of admission to neonatal intensive care units), neonatal intraventricular hemorrhage, and perinatal death are higher in women with chronic hypertension with superimposed preeclampsia compared with women who do not develop this complication.

Chappell LC, Seed PT, Briley AL, Kelly FJ, Lee R, Hunt BJ, et al. Effect of antioxidants on the occurrence of pre-eclampsia in women at increased risk: a randomised trial. Lancet. 1999;354:810-6. UI: 99413732

Chronic Renal Insufficiency in Pregnant Patients

- What is the most common life-threatening problem in pregnant patients with renal disease?
- What complications may affect outcome in patients with chronic renal disease who become pregnant?

Proteinuria > 300 mg/24 h during the first trimester in pregnant women with chronic hypertension is associated with a higher incidence of delivery of infants at < 35 weeks of gestation, birth weights low for gestational age, neonatal intraventricular hemorrhages, and more frequent admissions to neonatal intensive care units. Proteinuria may be an indication of underlying renal disease as a cause of the chronic hypertension and is a risk factor for adverse outcomes whether or not hypertension is controlled. Survival of infants of women with chronic renal insufficiency ranges between 70% and 100%, although prematurity and intrauterine growth retardation are common.

Women with preexisting nephropathy develop increased proteinuria and hypertension when pregnant. Although pregnant women with mild renal insufficiency may not develop impaired renal function as frequently as those with a lower GFR, there are few prospective data to substantiate this claim. Women with a serum creatinine concentration > 1.4 mg/dL in the first trimester have decreased fertility, and almost 50% may lose renal function during pregnancy or during the postpartum period. Women with a serum creatinine concentration > 2.0 mg/dL in the first trimester have a higher risk of pregnancy-associated progressive renal insufficiency. Similar outcomes occur in women with diabetic nephropathy. Flares of systemic lupus erythematosus may occur during pregnancy and the postpartum period and increase the risk of developing renal failure. Prednisone and azathioprine are used to treat these flares, but cyclophosphamide is teratogenic and must be avoided.

Most women with end-stage renal disease (ESRD) who are treated with dialysis are infertile, although pregnancy may occur in dialysis patients. Infant survival is improving, but only about 50% of women maintain the pregnancy to term (Hou). Many infants are premature or small for gestational age. However, 12% of women of childbearing age with a functioning renal transplant are able to conceive. Transplant recipients with a serum creatinine concentration < 2.0 mg/dL may have infants who are small for gestational age. Intensive dialysis has been used to attempt to maximize chances for successful delivery in pregnant women with renal insufficiency or ESRD, but there are no controlled studies to guide therapy.

KEY POINTS

- Hypertension is the most common life-threatening problem in pregnant patients with renal disease.
- Proteinuria in pregnant patients with chronic hypertension is a risk factor for adverse outcomes, whether or not hypertension is controlled.
- Women with a serum creatinine concentration > than 1.4 mg/dL in the first trimester have decreased fertility and may experience increased renal insufficiency during pregnancy or during the postpartum period.
- Women with a serum creatinine concentration > 2.0 mg/dL in the first trimester have an increased risk of pregnancy-associated progressive renal insufficiency.
- All pregnant women with a decreased glomerular filtration rate are at risk of developing preeclampsia and worsening renal function and should seek counseling prior to conceiving.
- The majority of women with end-stage renal disease who require dialysis are infertile. This may be reversible following successful transplantation.

Hou S. Pregnancy in chronic renal insufficiency and end-stage renal disease. Am J Kidney Dis. 1999;33:235-52. UI: 99146239

Acute Renal Failure in Pregnant Patients

- What are the causes of acute renal failure in pregnant patients?

Prerenal azotemia and urinary tract obstruction should be considered in all pregnant women with acute renal failure. Although urinary tract obstruction is rare, it may be difficult to diagnose because of the physiologic hydronephrosis of pregnancy. Acute renal failure in pregnancy is associated with abruptio placentae, septic abortion, severe preeclampsia, amniotic fluid embolism, and retained fetus. Acute renal failure in pregnancy is usually due to acute tubular necrosis or acute cortical necrosis. Anuria and hematuria, or the persistence of oliguria or anuria for more than 1 week, suggest cortical necrosis. The prognosis for recovery of renal function in patients with acute cortical necrosis is poor.

Postpartum acute renal failure is a rare but serious complication that can occur from several days to 10 weeks after delivery. Findings include hypertension, renal insufficiency, and microangiopathic hemolytic anemia. The syndrome is related to the thrombotic microangiopathies, thrombotic thrombo-\cytopenic purpura, and the hemolytic–uremic syndrome. A peripheral blood smear that shows signs of microangiopathic hemolytic anemia in the setting of thrombocytopenia and acute renal failure after delivery is diagnostic. Patients have been treated with plasma exchange, but renal failure often persists in survivors.

Self-Assessment Test

General Instructions

This self-assessment test contains one-best-answer multiple-choice questions. Please read these directions carefully before answering the questions.

The American College of Physicians–American Society of Internal Medicine designates MKSAP 12 Nephrology for a maximum of 10 hours in Category 1 credit towards the American Medical Association Physician's Recognition Award. Each physician should claim only those hours of credit that he/she actually spent in the educational activity.

Separate answer sheets are provided for each section of the MKSAP program. Please use one of these answer sheets to complete the Nephrology self-assessment test. Indicate in Section I on the answer sheet the actual credit hours you spend, up to the maximum listed above. If the hours spent are less than the maximum credit hours, you will be awarded credit hours for only the hours spent.

To have your scores included in the norm tables, submit your answer sheets to ACT, the test scoring agency by September 14, 2001. Performance reports will be mailed at the beginning of October 2001. Computer scoring will continue after the scoring deadlines until June 30, 2003, and you may submit your answer sheets at any time during this extended period.

Answers and Critiques

Answers, critiques, and bibliographies for these multiple-choice questions will be published with Part C, Book 6 of this program.

Directions

*Each of the numbered items or incomplete statements is followed by answers or by completions of the statement. Select the **ONE** lettered answer or completion that is **BEST** in each case.*

Item 1
A 20-year-old woman is evaluated during the third trimester of an otherwise uneventful first pregnancy because of right calf tenderness. Medical history is unremarkable. On physical examination, she is anxious, afebrile, and slightly tachypneic. Her respiratory rate is 16/min, and blood pressure is 105/75 mm Hg. Her abdomen is slightly tender. Her right calf is tender, but no venous cord is palpable. Homan's sign is negative.

Laboratory studies:

Hematocrit	31%
Leukocyte count	9000/µL; normal differential
Platelet count	220,000/µL
Blood urea nitrogen	5 mg/dL
Serum creatinine	0.6 mg/dL
Serum sodium	132 meq/L
Serum potassium	3.9 meq/L
Serum chloride	95 meq/L
Serum bicarbonate	20 meq/L
Arterial oxygen saturation	98%
Urinalysis	pH 6.0, specific gravity 1.020; dipstick negative; normal microscopic examination

Which of the following clinical scenarios is most likely, based on this patient's serum electrolyte values?

(A) Acute respiratory alkalosis secondary to a possible pulmonary embolism
(B) Metabolic acidosis due to a gastrointestinal disorder
(C) Hyperchloremic metabolic acidosis caused by renal tubular acidosis
(D) Normal electrolyte values in a pregnant woman

Item 2
A 68-year-old man has a 10-year history of hypertension, hypercholesterolemia treated with lovastatin, and intermittent claudication diagnosed 2 years ago. Despite treatment with β-blockers and diuretics, his blood pressure readings are typically 180/100–105 mm Hg and have never reached the goal of 140/90 mm Hg when measured in his physician's office. His serum creatinine concentration is 1.6 mg/dL. Enalapril, 10 mg daily, is started, and his blood pressure falls to 160/100 mm Hg. The dose of enalapril is subsequently increased to 20 mg daily.

The patient is seen 2 weeks later. On physical examination, his pulse rate is 98/min and regular and blood pressure is 130/70 mm Hg without orthostatic changes. There are no signs of volume overload. An epigastric bruit is heard on abdominal examination. His abdomen is nontender, and there are no enlarged organs. Popliteal pulses are intact, but the pedal pulses are decreased. There is no discoloration of the toes or pedal edema.

Laboratory studies:

Blood urea nitrogen	80 mg/dL
Serum creatinine	3.2 mg/dL
Serum sodium	135 meq/L
Serum potassium	5.2 meq/L
Serum chloride	99 meq/L
Serum bicarbonate	20 meq/L
Urinalysis	Specific gravity 1.016; trace protein, no blood, ketones, or glucose; normal microscopic examination

Which of the following is the most appropriate first step in managing this patient's acute renal failure?

(A) Discontinue enalapril; measure serum potassium and creatinine levels
(B) Discontinue the β-blocker; measure serum potassium and creatinine levels
(C) Discontinue lovastatin; measure the serum creatinine level
(D) Administer intravenous normal saline
(E) Obtain emergent renal arteriography

Item 3
A 77-year-old woman is evaluated because of dysuria, urinary frequency, pyuria, and fever. On physical examination, the patient weighs 54 kg (119 lb). Her temperature is 38.0 °C (100.4 °F). The remainder of her physical examination is normal. Her baseline serum creatinine value is 1.2 mg/dL. Urine culture grows greater than 100,000 colonies of *Escherichia coli*. You diagnose cystitis and prescribe trimethoprim-sulfamethoxazole orally twice daily for 7 days. On day 4 of treatment, the patient feels well, has no fever or urinary symptoms, and has no erythrocytes or leukocytes in

her urine. However, her serum creatinine value is now 1.8 mg/dL.

Which of the following statements is correct regarding her baseline serum creatinine value?

(A) The serum creatinine value of 1.2 mg/dL represents a normal glomerular filtration rate (GFR)
(B) The serum creatinine value of 1.2 mg/dL represents a GFR of less than 50% of normal
(C) Because of changes in the catabolism of creatinine in older persons, the serum creatinine value cannot be used to estimate the GFR in this patient
(D) Because of the effects of aging on renal function, this patient has an abnormally low GFR regardless of her serum creatinine value

Item 4
For the patient in the preceding question, which of the following is the most likely cause of the increase in her serum creatinine value from 1.2 mg/dL to 1.8 mg/dL?

(A) Acute interstitial nephritis due to trimethoprim-sulfamethoxazole
(B) Acute renal failure due to crystallization of sulfonamides in the renal tubules
(C) Bladder outlet obstruction
(D) Reduced tubular secretion of creatinine due to trimethoprim

Item 5
A 46-year-old white man comes to the emergency department because of cough and shortness of breath of several hours' duration. The patient, who smokes cigarettes, has had bilateral ankle and leg edema for 2 months. He has no history of heart disease.

On physical examination, his temperature is 36.9 °C (98.4 °F). His pulse rate is 102/min, respiratory rate is 26/min, and blood pressure is 150/82 mm Hg. He has periorbital edema. There is no neck vein distention. Cardiac examination discloses a normal S_1 and S_2 without murmurs or gallops. There are decreased breath sounds at the lung bases, but no crackles are heard. His abdomen is soft and nontender. There is 4+ edema of ankles and pretibial edema.

Laboratory studies:

Hematocrit	47%
Leukocyte count	9000/µL
Platelet count	325,000/µL
Plasma glucose	88 mg/dL
Blood urea nitrogen	24 mg/dL
Serum creatinine	1.2 mg/dL
Serum sodium	136 meq/L
Serum potassium	3.8 meq/L
Serum chloride	104 meq/L
Serum bicarbonate	26 meq/L
Plasma cholesterol	635 mg/dL
Serum albumin	1.6 g/dL

Arterial blood gas studies (patient breathing room air):

pH	7.48
P_{CO_2}	28 mm Hg
P_{O_2}	84 mm Hg
Bicarbonate	26 meq/L
Urinalysis	4+ protein, several erythrocytes/hpf

A chest radiograph shows basal atelectasis. An electrocardiogram reveals sinus tachycardia with no other abnormalities. A ventilation–perfusion lung scan is reported as indeterminate for pulmonary embolism.

Which of the following diagnostic studies should be done next?

(A) Echocardiography
(B) Doppler ultrasonography of the kidneys and renal vasculature
(C) Measurement of serum total complement and complement C3 concentrations
(D) Pulmonary function tests

Item 6
A 53-year-old man with a long history of chronic alcohol abuse comes to the emergency department because of a 3-week history of increasing weakness, anorexia, and a productive cough. On physical examination, the patient is thin and is obviously dyspneic. His pulse rate is 80/min and regular. Blood pressure is 130/70 mm Hg supine, falling to 120/65 mm Hg when he stands. There is a grade 2/6 systolic murmur and an S_3 gallop. Crackles are heard over the right hemithorax. Trace peripheral edema is noted.

Initial laboratory studies:

Blood urea nitrogen	12 mg/dL
Serum creatinine	1.0 mg/dL
Serum sodium	136 meq/L
Serum potassium	3.6 meq/L
Serum chloride	100 meq/L
Serum bicarbonate	22 meq/L

A chest radiograph shows an enlarged heart and a right middle lobe infiltrate or mass. The patient is hospitalized, and intravenous normal saline is begun at 100 mL/h. CT of the chest shows a lung lesion that is probably a mass. CT of the abdomen and pelvis shows an enlarged liver, several nodules suggesting metastatic lesions, and bilateral adrenal masses. The kidneys appear anatomically normal.

Laboratory studies on hospital day 4:

Blood urea nitrogen	8 mg/dL
Serum creatinine	1.0 mg/dL
Serum sodium	123 meq/L
Serum potassium	3.4 meq/L
Serum chloride	91 meq/L
Serum bicarbonate	20 meq/L
Serum uric acid	3.0 mg/dL
Urinary sodium	110 meq/L
Urinary potassium	40 meq/L
Urinary creatinine	85 mg/dL

Which of the following is the most likely cause of the decreasing serum sodium concentration in this patient?

(A) Extracellular fluid volume depletion
(B) Addison's disease
(C) Syndrome of inappropriate antidiuretic hormone secretion (SIADH)
(D) Cirrhosis
(E) Congestive heart failure

Item 7

A 28-year-old female cafeteria worker is evaluated because of an elevated blood pressure (approximately 160/105 mm Hg) for the past 2 to 3 months. The patient feels well. Her mother has hypertension and kidney disease, and a maternal aunt is currently on hemodialysis because of renal failure.

On physical examination, her height is 152 cm (62 in), and weight is 66 kg (145 lb). Her blood pressure is 166/106 mm Hg both seated and standing. The remainder of the examination is normal.

Laboratory studies:

Serum creatinine	0.8 mg/dL
Serum sodium	140 meq/L
Serum potassium	5.0 meq/L
Serum chloride	102 meq/L
Serum bicarbonate	25 meq/L
Serum thyroid-stimulating hormone	Normal
Urinalysis	Normal

An electrocardiogram is normal.

Which of the following diagnostic studies is most likely to provide information regarding the cause of her hypertension?

(A) Captopril-stimulated renal scan
(B) 24-Hour urine determination for vanillylmandelic acid
(C) Renal ultrasonography
(D) Plasma renin activity and aldosterone determinations

Item 8

A 50-year-old man underwent perineal prostatectomy 1 day ago for clinically localized prostate cancer. The patient has mild hypertension that is well controlled with diltiazem. He is otherwise healthy, and preoperative renal function was normal. A Foley catheter was placed preoperatively. The patient was in the dorsal lithotomy position for almost 6 hours and received approximately 3 L of lactated Ringer's solution perioperatively with a concomitant urine output of 568 mL. There was no significant decrease in mean arterial pressure or other notable events during the procedure. He tolerated the procedure well with minimal blood loss. However, he began to have decreasing urine output postoperatively. Four hours after the procedure, his urine output decreased to 10 mL/h. The catheter was flushed and was found to be working correctly. Two fluid boluses of 500 mL of normal saline were administered, but oliguria continued.

On physical examination today, the patient is responsive. His temperature is 36.8 °C (98.2 °F). His pulse rate is 95/min supine and 110/min sitting, respiratory rate is 18/min, and blood pressure is 132/85 mm Hg supine and 120/78 mm Hg sitting. His neck is supple, and no jugular venous distention is evident. His chest is clear. There is a systolic ejection murmur heard best at the left sternal border, but no gallop is heard. His abdomen is soft, distended, and nontender with infrequent bowel sounds. There is no peripheral edema.

Laboratory studies (immediately after surgery):

Blood urea nitrogen	20 mg/dL
Serum creatinine	2.2 mg/dL
Serum sodium	142 meq/L
Serum potassium	5.8 meq/L
Serum chloride	103 meq/L
Serum bicarbonate	19 meq/L
Serum calcium	7.0 mg/dL
Serum phosphorus	5.9 mg/dL

Laboratory studies (2 hours postoperatively):

Blood urea nitrogen	23 mg/dL
Serum creatinine	2.7 mg/dL
Serum sodium	146 meq/L
Serum potassium	6.9 meq/L
Serum chloride	106 meq/L
Serum bicarbonate	14 meq/L
Urinalysis	Specific gravity 1.025; trace protein, large blood, no glucose; muddy brown casts and cellular debris
Urinary sodium	32 meq/L

Electrocardiogram shows sinus tachycardia and peaked T waves.

Which of the following is the most likely diagnosis?

(A) Rhabdomyolysis
(B) Urinary tract obstruction
(C) Acute interstitial nephritis
(D) Rapidly progressive glomerulonephritis
(E) Prerenal azotemia

Item 9
A 31-year-old woman who has had type 1 diabetes mellitus since she was 3 years old now has anasarca, proliferative diabetic retinopathy, and peripheral sensory neuropathy. Her blood pressure is 143/90 mm Hg, and her serum creatinine is 2.1 mg/dL (serum creatinine was 1.4 mg/dL 1 year ago).

Which of the following 24-hour urinary values is most likely to be found?

(A) Protein of 6500 mg/24 h
(B) Protein of 800 mg/24 h
(C) Protein of 67 mg/24 h
(D) Albumin of 112 mg/24 h

Item 10
A 48-year-old man comes to your office because of a weight gain of 15.5 kg (34 lb) over the last 3 weeks. He has massive swelling of his feet and legs and reports swelling around his eyes in the morning and stiffness of his hands upon arising. Medical history is unremarkable.

On physical examination, his temperature is 36.9 °C (98.4 °F). His pulse rate is 82/min and regular, respiratory rate is 14/min, and blood pressure is 140/90 mm Hg. Periorbital edema is present. There is no neck vein distention. His chest is clear. Cardiac examination is normal. His abdomen is soft and nontender. There is 4+ pitting edema to both thighs.

Laboratory studies:

Hematocrit	42%
Leukocyte count	8200/µL
Platelet count	186,000/µL
Plasma glucose	126 mg/dL
Blood urea nitrogen	18 mg/dL
Serum creatinine	0.9 mg/dL
Serum sodium	140 meq/L
Serum potassium	4.3 meq/L
Serum chloride	106 meq/L
Serum bicarbonate	25 meq/L
Plasma cholesterol	486 mg/dL
Plasma albumin	1.8 g/dL
Urinalysis	4+ protein, several erythrocytes/hpf, oval fat bodies

Which of the following is the most appropriate initial treatment of this patient's edema?

(A) Low-salt diet alone with a goal of losing 0.45–0.9 kg (1–2 lb) daily
(B) Low-salt diet and spironolactone with a goal of losing 1.8–2.2 kg (4–5 lb) daily
(C) Low-salt diet and furosemide with a goal of losing 0.45–0.9 kg (1–2 lb) daily
(D) Low-salt diet and furosemide with a goal of losing 1.8–2.2 kg (4–5 lb) daily

Item 11
If the proteinuria of the patient in the preceding question does not improve, which of the following is most appropriate for his hyperlipidemia?

(A) Therapy is not necessary, since the hyperlipidemia is not associated with an increased risk of atherosclerotic events
(B) Dietary therapy alone with a low-saturated-fat, low-cholesterol diet will usually normalize the plasma cholesterol level
(C) Therapy should be started with both a low-saturated-fat, low-cholesterol diet and a 3-hydroxy-3-methylglutaryl–coenzyme A (HMG–CoA) reductase inhibitor
(D) The lipoprotein(a) level should be measured; if elevated, therapy with a 3-hydroxy-3-methylglutaryl–coenzyme A (HMG–CoA) reductase inhibitor should be started

Item 12
A 35-year-old woman has a history of recurrent calcium-containing kidney stones over the past 5 years. A previous evaluation included a normal serum calcium concentration and 24-hour urinary calcium excretion rate. She is seen today because of another episode of right flank pain. A plain radiograph of the abdomen and pelvis shows a radiopaque kidney stone at the right ureteropelvic junction.

Laboratory studies:

Blood urea nitrogen	28 mg/dL
Serum creatinine	1.0 mg/dL
Serum sodium	138 meq/L
Serum potassium	3.3 meq/L
Serum chloride	110 meq/L
Serum bicarbonate	18 meq/L

Which of the following urine studies would be most likely to suggest the correct underlying disorder?

(A) Calcium:creatinine ratio
(B) Transtubular potassium gradient
(C) pH

(D) Fractional excretion of sodium
(E) Urine culture with special instructions to maintain the culture for at least 1 week

Item 13
A 56-year-old woman is referred to you because of hypertension and hyperlipidemia. She had a thyroidectomy many years ago and has been on thyroid replacement therapy for more than 15 years. Four months ago, she was evaluated by her primary care physician because of fatigue. Multiple blood pressure readings at that time averaged 146/104 mm Hg. Plasma cholesterol was 312 mg/dL, and serum triglycerides were 268 mg/dL; other routine laboratory studies were normal.

A low-salt, low-saturated-fat diet was prescribed, but her blood pressure and hyperlipidemia did not improve. Renal duplex ultrasonography showed a normal-sized right kidney with a 60% stenosis and a normal left kidney and left renal artery. Plasma renin activity was suppressed at < 1 ng/L per hour. Plasma catecholamines were slightly elevated at 759 ng/L. Renal angiography was suggested, but the patient asked for a second opinion prior to having this study done.

On your physical examination, her height is 155 cm (61 in), and weight is 75 kg (165 lb). Pulse rate is 60/min, and blood pressure is 158/110 mm Hg both seated and standing. Funduscopic examination shows grade II hypertensive changes without hemorrhage, exudates, or papilledema. A thyroidectomy scar is present. There are no carotid or peripheral bruits. Cardiopulmonary examination is normal. Her abdomen is obese; there are no masses, bruits, or enlarged organs. Trace bilateral nonpitting pedal edema is noted.

Laboratory studies:

Plasma glucose	111 mg/dL
Blood urea nitrogen	22 mg/dL
Serum creatinine	0.9 mg/dL
Serum sodium	140 meq/L
Serum potassium	4.8 meq/L
Serum chloride	99 meq/L
Serum bicarbonate	28 meq/L
Serum calcium	9.6 mg/dL
Serum phosphorus	4.1 mg/dL

A chest radiograph and electrocardiogram are normal.

Which of the following is most appropriate at this time?

(A) Begin diuretic therapy
(B) Proceed with renal angiography
(C) Order thyroid-stimulating hormone determination
(D) Order 24-hour urine determination for vanillylmandelic acid; begin β-blocker therapy

Item 14
A 23-year-old woman comes to the emergency department because of nausea and back pain. HIV infection was diagnosed 2 months ago. Her serum creatinine concentration at that time was 0.6 mg/dL. Highly active antiretroviral therapy (HAART) with stavudine, delavirdine, and indinavir was started 3 weeks ago.

On physical examination, the patient is oriented. Her supine pulse rate is 98/min and regular, and blood pressure is 120/70 mm Hg without orthostatic changes. Her chest is clear, and no cardiac murmur or gallop is audible. Abdominal examination is normal. Left flank tenderness and moderate bilateral lower extremity edema are present.

Laboratory studies:

Blood urea nitrogen	80 mg/dL
Serum creatinine	4.7 mg/dL
Serum sodium	147 meq/L
Serum potassium	5.2 meq/L
Serum chloride	100 meq/L
Serum bicarbonate	18 meq/L
Urinalysis	Specific gravity 1.016; moderate blood, trace protein, trace ketones, no glucose; 7–10 erythrocytes/hpf; crystals and tubular cell casts, no erythrocyte casts

Which of the following is the most appropriate next step in this patient's care?

(A) Discontinue indinavir
(B) Administer captopril
(C) Schedule dialysis
(D) Administer sodium polystyrene sulfonate (Kayexalate)
(E) Discontinue stavudine

Item 15
A 54-year-old man is evaluated because of new-onset proteinuria detected by dipstick discovered during an insurance examination. On physical examination in your office, he weighs 81 kg (178 lb), and his blood pressure is 154/90 mm Hg. The remainder of his physical examination is normal.

Laboratory studies:

Serum creatinine	1.1 mg/dL
Urinary volume	1020 mL/24 h
Urinary creatinine	910 mg/24 h
Urinary protein	1250 mg/24 h
Creatinine clearance	62 mL/min

Which of the following statements is correct regarding the 24-hour urine collection?

(A) The 24-hour urinary protein is consistent with nephrotic-range proteinuria
(B) The creatinine clearance is inaccurate because the 24-hour urine collection is incomplete
(C) The creatinine clearance is inaccurate because the presence of proteinuria interferes with the urinary creatinine determination
(D) The 24-hour urine collection is accurate as evidenced by the fact that most adults excrete 900 to 1000 mg of creatinine daily

Item 16
A 42-year-old woman comes to your office for a routine evaluation. She received multiple transfusions 20 years earlier after an automobile accident. Over the last year, her serum creatinine level has risen from 1.0 mg/dL to 2.3 mg/dL.

On physical examination, her temperature is normal. Her pulse rate is 82/min, respiratory rate is 12/min, and blood pressure is 160/98 mm Hg. Heart sounds are normal, and her chest is clear. Mild hepatosplenomegaly is present. There is a petechial purpuric rash on her lower extremities; no edema is present.

Laboratory studies:

Complete blood count	Normal
Plasma glucose	Normal
Serum electrolytes	Normal
Serum complement:	
C3	Borderline low normal
C4	Reduced
CH_{50}	Reduced (25%)
Urinalysis	Many erythrocytes/hpf; erythrocyte casts
24-Hour urinary protein	3.5 g/24 h

Which of the following additional laboratory studies are most appropriate?

(A) Assays for antineutrophil cytoplasmic antibodies (ANCA) and anti–glomerular basement membrane (anti-GBM) antibodies
(B) Serum protein electrophoresis and urine immunoelectrophoresis
(C) Antistreptolysin O titer and antihyaluronidase assay
(D) Cryoglobulin determination and serologic tests for hepatitis C

Item 17
A 28-year-old pregnant woman with a 5-year history of proteinuria associated with focal and segmental glomerulosclerosis is seen 2 months after her last menstrual period. Five years ago, her serum creatinine concentration was 1.0 mg/dL and her creatinine clearance was 80 mL/min. Three years ago, her serum creatinine concentration was 1.4 mg/dL. She was treated with fosinopril with good blood pressure control, but the drug was discontinued 1 month ago, and methyldopa was started. On physical examination, she has gained 2.7 kg (6 lb). Her blood pressure is 135/88 mm Hg. She has trace pedal edema.

Laboratory studies:

Blood urea nitrogen	28 mg/dL
Serum creatinine	2.2 mg/dL
Serum uric acid	5.1 mg/dL
Urinalysis	4+ protein

Which of the following statements about this patient's course is correct?

(A) She is not at high risk for developing preeclampsia
(B) She is not at high risk for a premature birth
(C) She has a 1% to 2% risk of developing more severe renal insufficiency
(D) Her fetus is at risk for intrauterine growth retardation

Item 18
A 62-year-old male engineer is referred to you because of his difficult-to-control hypertension. High blood pressure was first noted 10 months ago and has not responded to increasing doses of amlodipine, losartan, and hydrochlorothiazide/triamterene. He has no history of cardiovascular or renal disease. Renal function studies, urinalysis, and renal scan obtained by his referring physician were normal.

On physical examination, his height is 180 cm (72 in), and weight is 82 kg (180 lb). Blood pressure is 170/105 mm Hg seated and standing. Funduscopic examination shows grade II hypertensive retinopathy. Cardiopulmonary examination is normal. Abdominal examination discloses no masses, bruits, or enlarged organs. Trace bilateral pedal edema is noted.

Laboratory studies:

Plasma glucose	89 mg/dL
Blood urea nitrogen	16 mg/dL
Serum creatinine	0.7 mg/dL
Serum sodium	140 meq/L
Serum potassium	3.2 meq/L
Serum chloride	100 meq/L
Serum bicarbonate	27 meq/L
Serum thyroid-stimulating hormone	Normal
Urinalysis	Normal

Which of the following would be most appropriate at this time?

(A) Add potassium chloride to his current regimen to correct his hypokalemia; no additional diagnostic studies are indicated
(B) Discontinue losartan and hydrochlorothiazide/triamterene for 2 weeks; obtain a 24-hour urine specimen for sodium, potassium, and aldosterone excretion during oral salt-loading
(C) Discontinue losartan; order a captopril-stimulated renal scan
(D) Discontinue losartan and hydrochlorothiazide/triamterene for 2 weeks; obtain a serum aldosterone determination

Items 19, 20
A 58-year-old woman is hospitalized because of acute renal failure. One week ago, acute B-cell lymphoblastic leukemia was diagnosed. Today, 3 days before she was to begin chemotherapy, she came to the office for examination and to receive a prescription for allopurinol. She was asymptomatic but stated that her urine output had been decreasing for 24 to 36 hours.

On physical examination, her temperature was 37.3°C (99.2 °F). Her pulse rate was 100/min and regular, respiratory rate was 14/min and regular, and blood pressure was 120/60 mm Hg without orthostatic changes. Diffuse lymphadenopathy was noted. Cardiovascular examination was normal. The liver and spleen were not enlarged, and there was no abdominal bruit. Neurologic examination was normal. Distal pulses were strong and present bilaterally. There was 1+ pedal edema.

Laboratory studies:

Hematocrit	29%
Leukocyte count	24,500/µL; 52% lymphocytes, 5% eosinophils, 1% neutrophils, 3% monocytes, 2% basophils, 37% large undetermined cells
Platelet count	99,000/µL
Prothrombin time	Normal
Blood urea nitrogen	43 mg/dL
Serum creatinine	3.0 mg/dL
Serum sodium	144 meq/L
Serum potassium	5.6 meq/L
Serum chloride	100 meq/L
Serum bicarbonate	15 meq/L
Serum calcium	9.2 mg/dL
Serum phosphorus	4.3 mg/dL
Serum uric acid	19.3 mg/dL
Serum aspartate aminotransferase	40 U/L
Serum alanine aminotransferase	35 U/L
Serum amylase	49 U/L
Serum bilirubin	0.9 mg/dL
Urinalysis	Specific gravity 1.007, pH 5.0; 1+ protein, no blood, ketones, or glucose; rare leukocytes/hpf, several granular cell casts, no leukocyte or erythrocyte casts
Urinary sodium	46 meq/L
Urinary osmolality	208 mosm/kg H_2O
Urinary creatinine	25 mg/dL
Urinary uric acid	37 mg/dL

The patient is hospitalized. A 24-hour urine collection after admission to the hospital showed a volume of 355 mL. Urine culture showed no growth.

Item 19
Which of the following statements is correct regarding acute renal failure in this patient?

(A) The fractional excretion of sodium suggests prerenal azotemia
(B) The urinary uric acid:urinary creatinine ratio suggests that uric acid–mediated injury underlies the pathologic process
(C) The course is consistent with rhabdomyolysis
(D) The absence of hyperphosphatemia rules out the diagnosis of tumor lysis syndrome
(E) Tumor lysis syndrome does not develop unless antineoplastic therapy is administered

Item 20
Which of the following is <u>contraindicated</u> in the initial management of this patient?

(A) Ultrasonography or non-contrast-enhanced CT of the abdomen
(B) Administration of allopurinol
(C) Dialysis as needed
(D) Renal arteriography

Item 21
A 42-year-old man is evaluated because of right renal colic and microhematuria. He has had three previous episodes of calcium nephrolithiasis. Diagnostic studies show a 4-mm calcified stone in the middle right ureter.

Which of the following laboratory test results is not a risk factor for calcium nephrolithiasis?

(A) Urinary calcium of 315 mg/24 h
(B) Serum uric acid of 10.5 mg/dL
(C) Urinary citrate of 100 mg/24 h (normal 300–700 mg/24 h)
(D) Urinary oxalate of 72 mg/24 h (normal < 40 mg/24 h)
(E) Serum calcium of 11 mg/dL and serum phosphorus of 2.1 mg/dL

Item 22
A 54-year-old black American man is found to have idiopathic nephrotic syndrome with normal blood urea nitrogen and serum creatinine levels. A renal biopsy has been recommended to determine the histopathologic diagnosis and potential course of therapy. Before undergoing the biopsy, the patient wishes to know what is most likely to be found and whether it is treatable.

Which of the following is the most appropriate answer to this patient's question?

(A) Membranous nephropathy is the most likely diagnosis, and immunosuppressive therapy is successful in up to 50% of patients
(B) Minimal change disease is the most likely diagnosis because of the normal blood urea nitrogen and serum creatinine levels, and treatment with glucocorticoids will likely induce a remission of the proteinuria
(C) Focal glomerulosclerosis is the most likely diagnosis because it is the most common pattern of idiopathic nephrotic syndrome in black Americans, and treatment with a prolonged course of glucocorticoids is successful in up to 50% of patients
(D) AL amyloidosis is the most likely diagnosis in patients over 50 years of age, and treatment includes chemotherapy

Item 23
A 26-year-old woman comes to the emergency department because of paresthesias, perioral numbness, and generalized weakness. She denies use of any medications. Her blood pressure is 120/88 mm Hg, and physical examination is unremarkable.

Laboratory studies:

Blood urea nitrogen	15 mg/dL
Serum creatinine	1.2 mg/dL
Serum sodium	136 meq/L
Serum potassium	2.8 meq/L
Serum chloride	90 meq/L
Serum bicarbonate	38 meq/L
Urine pH	5.8
Urinary sodium	18 meq/L
Urinary potassium	20 meq/L
Urinary chloride	5 meq/L
Urinary calcium:creatinine ratio	0.3

Which of the following is the most likely diagnosis?

(A) Bartter's syndrome
(B) Surreptitious vomiting
(C) Gitelman's syndrome
(D) Hypokalemic periodic paralysis
(E) Licorice ingestion

Item 24
A 48-year-old woman was found to have primary hypertension 6 months ago. Despite a trial of lifestyle modifications, her blood pressure remained elevated at about 158/96 mm Hg. Therapy with amlodipine, 5 mg daily, was begun.

The patient returns for a follow-up visit 6 weeks after beginning amlodipine. Several blood pressures readings in your office average 152/92 mm Hg. She has also noted progressive ankle edema since therapy was begun.

Which of the following is most appropriate at this time?

(A) No change in therapy; return for a follow-up visit in 3 to 6 weeks
(B) Change to another antihypertensive agent and increase the dose until her blood pressure is < 140/90 mm Hg
(C) Increase the amlodipine to 10 mg daily
(D) Prescribe a low-salt diet and support hose for control of localized edema

Items 25, 26
A 59-year-old male smoker is hospitalized after sustaining an acute anterior wall myocardial infarction. He has a 16-year history of type 2 diabetes mellitus and hypertension. Current medications are metformin and diltiazem.

On physical examination, his temperature is 37.8 °C (101.8 °F). His pulse rate is 75/min, respiratory rate is 18/min, and blood pressure is 145/85 mm Hg. Mucous membranes are dry, and moderate jugular venous distention is present. His chest is clear, and no murmurs or gallops are heard. His abdomen is soft, nontender, and nondistended. There is no sacral or lower extremity edema.

Laboratory studies (on admission):

Hemoglobin	12.0 g/dL
Hematocrit	38%
Leukocyte count	8000/µL
Platelet count	256,000/µL
Blood urea nitrogen	22 mg/dL
Serum creatinine	1.6 mg/dL
Serum sodium	140 meq/L
Serum potassium	5.1 meq/L

Serum chloride	105 meq/L
Serum bicarbonate	26 meq/L
Serum calcium	9.0 mg/dL
Serum magnesium	1.6 mg/dL
Serum phosphorus	2.9 mg/dL
Urinalysis	pH 6.0; 1+ protein, 1+ glucose, no blood or ketones; no formed elements on microscopic examination

The patient is scheduled to undergo coronary angiography in the morning.

Which of the following is the most effective preventive measure to reduce the risk of contrast nephropathy in this patient?

(A) Administer intravenous half-normal saline and intravenous furosemide at the time of angiography
(B) Administer intravenous half-normal saline and intravenous mannitol at the time of angiography
(C) Administer intravenous half-normal saline before performing angiography
(D) Limit the dose of intravenous contrast to < 0.5 mL/kg/h and administer concurrent intravenous dopamine at the time of angiography
(E) Discontinue the diltiazem

Item 26

In the previous patient, angiography revealed two lesions, one in the proximal left anterior descending artery and one in the first diagonal artery. Both were treated with angioplasty and stent placement.

Thirty-six hours after the procedure, the patient's laboratory values were:

Blood urea nitrogen	33 mg/dL
Serum creatinine	2.9 mg/dL
Serum sodium	143 meq/L
Serum potassium	5.3 meq/L
Serum chloride	110 meq/L
Serum bicarbonate	24 meq/L
Urinalysis	Specific gravity 1.015; trace protein, trace glucose, no blood; few hyaline casts on microscopic examination

Which of the following is indicated to reduce the morbidity associated with the patient's contrast nephropathy?

(A) Monitor; begin renal replacement therapy if indicated
(B) Administer intravenous half-normal saline and intravenous dopamine for 24 hours
(C) Administer intravenous half-normal saline
(D) Begin dialysis to clear residual contrast as soon as possible
(E) Discontinue the diltiazem

Item 27

Three months ago, a 47-year-old woman experienced mild right flank pain for several hours associated with gross hematuria. Since then, she has had several episodes of gross painless hematuria. There has been no fever, chills, dysuria, or weight loss.

On physical examination, she is alert and in no distress. Temperature is 36.6 °C (97.9 °F). Her pulse rate is 69/min, and blood pressure is 137/89 mm Hg. The examination is normal except for moderate obesity and slight costovertebral angle tenderness.

Laboratory studies:

Serum creatinine	0.8 mg/dL
Serum sodium	140 meq/L
Serum potassium	3.8 meq/L
Serum chloride	102 meq/L
Serum bicarbonate	26 meq/L
Urinalysis	pH 4.5; 3+ heme, no protein; 40–50 erythrocytes, occasional leukocytes/hpf; no bacteria, no crystals

A plain radiograph of the abdomen and pelvis is normal. Spiral CT without contrast shows a bright 1.5-cm object in the right renal pelvis with slight right hydronephrosis. The kidneys are 12 cm in length with normal parenchymal thickness.

Which of the following is the most likely diagnosis?

(A) Calcium oxalate stone in the right renal pelvis
(B) Transitional cell carcinoma of the bladder
(C) Uric acid stone in the right renal pelvis
(D) Analgesic nephropathy
(E) Chronic pyelonephritis

Item 28

A 68-year-old man is evaluated because of progressive swelling of his lower extremities. He has no prior history of cardiovascular or renal disease.

On physical examination, his temperature is normal. His pulse rate is 68/min, respiratory rate is 12/min, and blood pressure is 138/82 mm Hg. His chest is clear. Cardiac examination reveals an S_4 gallop. Abdominal examination discloses a palpable spleen tip and an enlarged liver. There is 4+ bilateral pedal edema.

Laboratory studies:

Complete blood count	Normal
Plasma glucose	Normal
Blood urea nitrogen	25 mg/dL
Serum creatinine	1.8 mg/dL
Serum electrolytes	Normal
Urinalysis	3+ to 4+ protein, trace heme
24-Hour urinary albumin	5.6 g/24 h

An electrocardiogram shows low voltage but no other abnormalities. A chest radiograph is normal. Serum protein electrophoresis discloses an abnormal monoclonal protein in the gamma region, which on immunoelectrophoresis is found to be 2.3 g of IgG lambda.

Which of the following is the most likely cause of this patient's renal insufficiency?

(A) Membranous nephropathy
(B) Myeloma cast nephropathy
(C) Amyloidosis
(D) Light chain deposition disease

Item 29
A 50-year-old woman with a long history of type 1 diabetes mellitus develops an upper respiratory tract infection and fever. She then develops polyuria and thirst and comes to the emergency department. On physical examination, her temperature is 38.3 °C (101.0 °F). Her blood pressure is 110/70 mm Hg supine and 90/65 mm Hg seated. Funduscopic examination shows diabetic retinopathy. Cardiopulmonary examination is normal. Abdominal examination reveals some right upper quadrant tenderness. There is 1+ peripheral edema.

Laboratory studies:

Plasma glucose	1200 mg/dL
Blood urea nitrogen	38 mg/dL
Serum creatinine	2.1 mg/dL
Serum sodium	124 meq/L
Serum potassium	4.1 meq/L
Serum chloride	90 meq/L
Serum bicarbonate	10 meq/L

A diagnosis of ketoacidosis is made. Along with insulin, isotonic saline is infused to restore extracellular fluid volume, and potassium chloride is given to correct the hypokalemia that later developed. No free water or additional solute was administered.

This patient's serum sodium concentration is most likely to be which of the following after her plasma glucose has been restored to 120 mg/dL?

(A) Less than 120 meq/L
(B) About 124 meq/L
(C) 135 to 145 meq/L
(D) Greater than 149 meq/L

Item 30
A 55-year-old male lawyer has progressive chronic renal insufficiency due to type 2 diabetic nephropathy and hypertension. His creatinine clearance is 23 mL/min, and his serum creatinine is 3.1 mg/dL. He has just returned from an introductory educational session regarding dialysis and transplantation options, which was arranged by the consulting nephrologist. He asks your opinion about potential options.

Which of the following offers the best prognosis for this patient?

(A) Peritoneal dialysis
(B) Hemodialysis
(C) Renal transplantation
(D) Combined renal and pancreas transplantation

Item 31
A 53-year-old Chinese-American woman recently returned to the United States from a trip to China. Type 2 diabetes mellitus was diagnosed 4 months before the start of her trip. Because she was at her ideal weight, treatment with oral hypoglycemics was suggested, but she declined because she was "afraid of medicines." She was normotensive, and her serum creatinine concentration at the time of diagnosis was 0.7 mg/dL. There was no evidence of microalbuminuria. On her return to the United States, she saw her primary care physician for her regular checkup. Her physical examination was unchanged, but her serum creatinine concentration was 1.9 mg/dL. On questioning, she told her physician that she had started taking medications in China "to protect her kidneys." She is referred to you.

On physical examination, her temperature is 36.8 °C (98.2 °F). Her pulse rate is 88/min, respiratory rate is 14/min and regular, and blood pressure is 130/82 mm Hg without orthostatic changes. There is no rash and no neck vein distention. Her chest is clear. S_1 and S_2 are normal, and no gallops or murmurs are heard. Abdominal examination is normal. There is 1+ pedal edema. Distal pulses are present. Neurologic examination is normal.

Laboratory studies:

Hematocrit	28%
Leukocyte count	6500/µL; normal differential
Platelet count	299,000/µL
Blood urea nitrogen	34 mg/dL
Serum creatinine	1.9 mg/dL
Serum sodium	141 meq/L
Serum potassium	5.3 meq/L

Serum chloride	99 meq/L
Serum bicarbonate	21 meq/L
Serum bilirubin	0.9 mg/dL
Serum aspartate aminotransferase	Normal
Serum alanine aminotransferase	Normal
Serum amylase	Normal
Serum creatine kinase	Normal
Urinalysis	Specific gravity 1.007, pH 5.0; 1+ protein, no blood, ketones, or glucose; no erythrocytes, scant leukocytes/hpf, several granular casts, no erythrocyte or leukocyte casts
Urine culture	No growth

Which of the following is the most likely cause of the acute renal failure?

(A) Diabetic nephropathy
(B) IgA nephropathy
(C) Nephropathy due to Chinese herbs
(D) Prerenal azotemia

Item 32
A 34-year-old woman is referred from the emergency department because of bilateral foot and leg swelling. She recently was found to be infected with HIV.

On physical examination, her temperature is 36.7 °C (98.0 °F). Her pulse rate is 88/min, respiratory rate is 14/min, and blood pressure is 126/78 mm Hg. There is 2+ to 3+ pedal and ankle edema. The remainder of the physical examination is normal.

Laboratory studies:

Hematocrit	35%
Leukocyte count	5600/μL
Platelet count	345,000/μL
Blood urea nitrogen	22 mg/dL
Serum creatinine	1.6 mg/dL
Serum total complement	Normal
Antinuclear antibody	Negative
Antistreptolysin O	Negative
Antineutrophil cytoplasmic antibody	Negative
Urinalysis	4+ protein, 2+ heme; several erythrocytes/hpf, broad casts
24-Hour urinary protein	16 g/24 h

Which of the following diagnostic studies may help suggest the most likely cause of this patient's renal disorder prior to renal biopsy?

(A) Renal ultrasonography
(B) Intravenous pyelography
(C) Renal angiography
(D) Echocardiography

Item 33
A renal biopsy is performed on the patient in the preceding question and shows collapsing focal glomerulosclerosis with tubular microcyst formation.

In addition to highly active antiretroviral therapy (HAART) for the HIV infection, which of the following is the most appropriate therapy for this patient's renal disease?

(A) An angiotensin-converting enzyme inhibitor
(B) Pulse intravenous methylprednisolone
(C) A dihydropyridine calcium channel blocker
(D) Cyclophosphamide

Item 34
A 35-year-old man with chronic renal failure undergoes hemodialysis three times each week. His compliance has been poor, and he has missed his last dialysis treatment. He now comes to the emergency department because of weakness and nausea.

Laboratory studies:

Serum sodium	128 meq/L
Serum potassium	7.2 meq/L
Serum chloride	95 meq/L
Serum bicarbonate	15 meq/L

An electrocardiogram shows first-degree heart block, peaked T waves, and wide QRS complexes. While awaiting dialysis, he receives infusions of calcium gluconate, sodium bicarbonate, glucose, and insulin. He also receives inhaled albuterol and oral sodium polystyrene sulfonate (Kayexalate).

Which of these medications is <u>least</u> likely to reduce his serum potassium concentration?

(A) Albuterol
(B) Sodium bicarbonate
(C) Glucose and insulin
(D) Calcium gluconate
(E) Sodium polystyrene sulfonate (Kayexalate)

Item 35
A 29-year-old woman with type 1 diabetes mellitus is evaluated because of a 10-day history of urinary frequency, mild dysuria, and "slight fever." She has no history of chills, hematuria, renal stones, or flank pain. She reports that similar episodes have occurred once or twice yearly for the past 6 years. She previously treated herself with fluids and cran-

berry juice or went to an urgent care center, where she was told that she had cystitis and was given antibiotics. There is no family history of renal disease. Physical examination is normal.

Laboratory studies:

Hematocrit	39%
Serum creatinine	0.8 mg/dL
Serum sodium	139 meq/L
Serum potassium	4.0 meq/L
Serum chloride	100 meq/L
Serum bicarbonate	24 meq/L
Serum calcium	9.0 mg/dL
Serum albumin	2.8 g/dL
Urinalysis	pH 6.5; 2+ heme, trace protein, trace glucose; 5–10 erythrocytes, 40–50 leukocytes/hpf; many bacteria; leukocyte-esterase positive
Urine culture	> 100,000 colonies of *Proteus mirabilis*

A plain radiograph of the abdomen and pelvis shows an irregular calcified object measuring 3 × 5 cm overlying the right renal shadow. An intravenous pyelogram shows a branched calcified calculus occupying the upper half of the right renal collecting system with loss of renal parenchymal thickness of the right kidney. The left kidney is normal.

Which of the following stone diseases does this patient most likely have?

(A) Calcium oxalate stone
(B) Calcium phosphate and oxalate stones
(C) Uric acid stone
(D) Triple phosphate (struvite) stone

Item 36

A 48-year-old male renal transplant recipient is evaluated because of severe pain in his right great toe for the past 36 hours. He denies fever, chills, or other systemic symptoms. The patient had end-stage renal disease secondary to autosomal dominant polycystic kidney disease and received a successful renal transplant 2 years ago. His serum creatinine level has remained stable at 2.1 mg/dL on an immunosuppressive regimen of prednisone, 7.5 mg daily; azathioprine, 100 mg daily; and cyclosporine, 125 mg twice daily. The patient has a history of intermittent gout (documented by arthrocentesis), which has flared more frequently during the past 6 months.

On physical examination, his height is 165 cm (65 in) and weight is 72 kg (159 lb). His blood pressure is 138/88 mm Hg seated and standing. Examination is normal except for exquisite tenderness and erythema at the base of his right great toe.

Laboratory studies:

Complete blood count	Normal
Plasma glucose	111 mg/dL
Blood urea nitrogen	30 mg/dL
Serum creatinine	1.9 mg/dL
Serum sodium	138 meq/L
Serum potassium	4.8 meq/L
Serum chloride	101 meq/L
Serum bicarbonate	23 meq/L
Serum uric acid	10.1 mg/dL
Urinalysis	Normal

Which of the following is most appropriate for treating this patient's gout?

(A) Begin indomethacin, 25 mg to 50 mg three times daily, and allopurinol, 300 mg daily
(B) Begin colchicine; recommend subsequent allopurinol, 300 mg daily
(C) Increase prednisone to 30 mg daily with a tapering dose; recommend subsequent allopurinol, 300 mg daily
(D) Begin colchicine; recommend subsequent allopurinol, 100 mg daily, with a 50% to 75% reduction of his azathioprine dose

Items 37, 38

A 55-year-old woman was hospitalized because of fever and fatigue. Medical history revealed mitral valve prolapse and mild essential hypertension that has been well controlled with atenolol for the past 6 years. Blood cultures after admission grew viridans streptococci. A diagnosis of bacterial endocarditis was made, and intravenous gentamicin and ampicillin were begun. Serum creatinine on admission was 0.6 mg/dL. On day 8, the patient was discharged and placed on home intravenous therapy. Her serum creatinine on discharge was 0.7 mg/dL. On day 16 of therapy, her serum creatinine, drawn by the visiting nurse, was 2.2 mg/dL. She is readmitted to the hospital.

On physical examination on admission, temperature is 36.8 °C (98.2 °F). Her pulse rate is 87/min, respiratory rate is 12/min, and blood pressure is 167/98 mm Hg without orthostatic changes. Mucous membranes are moist, and there is no rash. There is no jugular venous distention. Her chest is clear. There is a soft systolic murmur at the apex, but no gallop is heard. Her abdomen is soft and nontender. Lower extremity pulses are 2+, and there is no sacral or lower extremity edema.

Laboratory studies:

Hemoglobin	11.6 g/dL
Hematocrit	35%

Leukocyte count	8500/μL; 65% neutrophils, 30% lymphocytes, 3% monocytes, 2% basophils
Platelet count	152,000/μL
Blood urea nitrogen	39 mg/dL
Serum creatinine	2.3 mg/dL
Serum sodium	143 meq/L
Serum potassium	5.5 meq/L
Serum chloride	109 meq/L
Serum bicarbonate	21 meq/L
Serum calcium	8.7 mg/dL
Serum phosphorus	4.7 mg/dL
Urinalysis	Specific gravity 1.011; trace protein, no blood or glucose; muddy granular casts but no erythrocyte or leukocyte casts; no bacteria
Urinary sodium	42 meq/L

Item 37
Which of the following is the most likely diagnosis?

(A) Prerenal azotemia
(B) Acute interstitial nephritis
(C) Aminoglycoside nephrotoxicity
(D) Rhabdomyolysis
(E) Glomerulonephritis associated with bacterial endocarditis

Item 38
For the patient in the preceding question, which of the following is most appropriate at this time?

(A) Begin intravenous methylprednisolone
(B) Begin intravenous normal saline with dopamine at 3 units/kg/min
(C) Discontinue gentamicin
(D) Alkalinize the urine with sodium bicarbonate

Item 39
Which of the following statements is correct regarding autosomal dominant polycystic kidney disease (ADPKD)?

(A) ADPKD is invariably associated with end-stage renal disease by the time patients are 50 years old
(B) ADPKD is more common in men than in women
(C) ADPKD is associated with hepatic cysts in up to 50% of patients as they age
(D) ADPKD is less common in black Americans than in other racial groups in the United States

Item 40
A 22-year-old female college student comes to your office because she developed dark urine after playing basketball. She denies joint symptoms or rash but does recall a sore throat about 1 week prior to the episode of dark urine. On physical examination, her blood pressure is normal, and there is no edema. The remainder of the examination is normal. Complete blood count, blood urea nitrogen, serum creatinine, serum electrolytes, and serum complement are also normal. Antinuclear antibody assay is negative. Urinalysis shows 1+ protein, many erythrocytes/hpf, and erythrocyte casts.

Which of the following is the most likely diagnosis?

(A) Poststreptococcal glomerulonephritis
(B) Lupus nephritis
(C) IgA nephropathy
(D) Sickle cell nephropathy

Item 41
A 24-year-old man is brought to the emergency department after being found unresponsive on the floor of his shower. He has a longstanding history of chronic schizophrenia and has required two previous hospitalizations for hyponatremia related to psychogenic water ingestion.

On physical examination, he is still unresponsive. He has bitten his tongue and may be postictal. His pulse rate is 100/min and regular, and blood pressure is 130/80 mm Hg. Physical examination is otherwise unremarkable.

Laboratory studies:

Blood urea nitrogen	12 mg/dL
Serum creatinine	0.8 mg/dL
Serum sodium	108 meq/L
Serum potassium	3.5 meq/L
Serum chloride	80 meq/L
Serum bicarbonate	16 meq/L

Which of the following is most appropriate for this patient?

(A) Hypertonic (3%) saline to increase the sodium concentration by 10 to 15 meq/L over several hours
(B) Hypertonic (3%) saline to increase the sodium concentration by 0.5 meq/h over 24 hours
(C) Parenteral furosemide and strict water restriction (< 200 mL/24 h)
(D) Normal saline, 2 L at 200 mL/h

Item 42
A 54-year-old male renal transplant recipient is evaluated because of headache, dizziness, and loss of balance. There is no history of loss of consciousness or seizures.

The patient has end-stage renal disease secondary to chronic glomerulonephritis. After a period of hemodialysis, he received a successful cadaveric renal transplant 13 months ago. His course was complicated by two bouts of acute rejection requiring intravenous methylprednisolone and muromonab CD3 (OKT3) therapy. After his first bout of rejection, he developed cytomegalovirus infection. Current medications are prednisone, cyclosporine, and azathioprine. His serum creatinine level has been stable on this regimen.

On physical examination, he appears well. Blood pressure is 142/86 mm Hg without orthostatic changes. Neurologic examination discloses mild nystagmus and a positive Romberg sign. Cardiopulmonary and abdominal examinations are normal. There is no peripheral lymphadenopathy.

MRI of the head shows a 3-cm lesion in the posterior fossa with a patent fourth ventricle. Biopsy of the mass shows that the lesion is a large cell lymphoma (non-Hodgkin's lymphoma).

Which of the following statements is correct regarding this patient's disorder?

(A) This disorder is much more common in renal transplant recipients than in heart transplant recipients because of the increased immunosuppressive therapy required
(B) This disorder is usually due to a Hodgkin's lymphoma of T-cell origin that develops in nodal rather than extranodal sites
(C) The appearance of this disorder is unrelated to the type of organ transplanted and the immunosuppressive therapy used
(D) This disorder appears to be related to B-cell proliferation induced by Epstein-Barr virus infection in patients who are receiving chronic immunosuppressive therapy

Item 43

A 63-year-old woman who has chronic inflammatory demyelinating polyneuropathy was started on intravenous immune globulin G (IgG) after having had no response to prolonged glucocorticoid therapy. Glucocorticoids were stopped 2 months ago. Her first dose of immune globulin G was 7 days ago, and she received four additional doses of 400 mg/kg, ending 2 days ago. She experienced headaches during some of the infusions and was treated with ibuprofen on the third and fourth days. She did not notice a change in her neurologic status after therapy. She contacts you today because of scanty urine output and discolored urine over the last 24 hours. The patient has no history of diabetes mellitus, hypertension, or renal disease.

On physical examination, her temperature is 37.2 °C (99.0 °F). Her pulse rate is 120/min, respiratory rate is 20/min, and blood pressure is 160/98 mm Hg. Scant crackles are auscultated, but no murmurs or gallops are heard. Abdominal examination is normal. There is 2+ peripheral edema. Neurologic examination shows severe distal lower extremity weakness, areflexia, and markedly diminished sensation.

Laboratory studies:

Blood urea nitrogen	30 mg/dL
Serum creatinine	2.7 mg/dL
Serum sodium	142 meq/L
Serum potassium	5.1 meq/L
Serum chloride	98 meq/L
Serum bicarbonate	16 meq/L
Urinalysis	Specific gravity 1.009; 1+ protein; 2–3 erythrocytes, 10 leukocytes/hpf; no erythrocyte or leukocyte casts
Urine culture	No growth

Which of the following is most appropriate at this time?

(A) Provide vigorous fluid repletion
(B) Prepare the patient for chronic dialysis
(C) Perform plasmapheresis
(D) Discontinue immune globulin G

Item 44

A 38-year-old man with chronic renal failure comes to the emergency department because of weakness, anorexia, and nausea. He has recently had increasing nausea and vomiting but has refused to begin dialysis despite your recommendation to do so. Physical examination discloses bibasilar crackles, a regular cardiac rhythm without gallops, no enlarged abdominal organs, and 2+ peripheral edema.

Laboratory studies:

Blood urea nitrogen	100 mg/dL
Serum creatinine	12.0 mg/dL
Serum sodium	135 meq/L
Serum potassium	5.2 meq/L
Serum chloride	80 meq/L
Serum bicarbonate	24 meq/L

Arterial blood gas studies (patient breathing room air):

pH	7.40
P_{CO_2}	37 mm Hg
Bicarbonate	22 meq/L

Which of the following best describes this patient's acid-base status?

(A) No acid-base abnormality
(B) Metabolic acidosis and respiratory alkalosis
(C) Metabolic acidosis and metabolic alkalosis
(D) Respiratory acidosis and respiratory alkalosis

Item 45
A 66-year-old male machinist is hospitalized for evaluation and management of azotemia. Prior to admission he had seen his primary care physician because of chronic sinusitis and headache. During his evaluation, his serum creatinine level was 3.9 mg/dL. Eight months ago, his serum creatinine level was 1.7 mg/dL. The patient denied a history of fever, chills, weight loss, other systemic symptoms, or exposure to any nephrotoxic drugs or contrast agents. He has a 15-year history of hypertension. Medications include verapamil, 240 mg daily, and aspirin, one tablet daily.

On physical examination on admission, his weight is 82 kg (181 lb). Temperature is normal. His blood pressure is 148/92 mm Hg supine and 128/84 mm Hg standing. A detailed examination is normal

Laboratory studies (on admission):

Hemoglobin	11.3 g/dL
Leukocyte count	Normal
Platelet count	Normal
Blood urea nitrogen	68 mg/dL
Serum creatinine	3.9 mg/dL
Serum sodium	136 meq/L
Serum potassium	3.9 meq/L
Serum chloride	100 meq/L
Serum bicarbonate	22 meq/L
Serum calcium	14.1 mg/dL
Serum phosphorus	4.2 mg/dL
Serum albumin	4.2 g/dL
Urinalysis	Specific gravity 1.009, pH 6.0, 1+ protein, no heme, no casts

A chest radiograph shows an interstitial infiltrate and a left paratracheal lymph node.

Treatment is begun with aggressive intravenous saline hydration followed by intravenous furosemide and subcutaneous calcitonin. The following morning, his serum creatinine level is 3.2 mg/dL, and his serum calcium level is 12.6 mg/dL. Additional laboratory test results show serum parathyroid hormone of 18 pg/mL (normal: 8 to 65 pg/mL), 1,25-dihydroxyvitamin D of 89 pg/mL (normal: 10 to 50 pg/mL), and normal serum and urine immunoelectrophoresis without a monoclonal M-spike.

Which of the following is most likely causing this patient's impaired renal function?

(A) Hyperparathyroidism
(B) Sarcoidosis
(C) Multiple myeloma kidney
(D) Metastatic lung cancer
(E) Wegener's granulomatosis

Item 46
Treatment is continued for the patient in the preceding question. By the third hospital day, his serum creatinine level has fallen to 2.1 mg/dL and his serum calcium level has decreased to 10.6 mg/dL. A paratracheal lymph node biopsy specimen shows six foci of histiocytes and giant cells. Stains for acid-fast bacilli and fungi are negative. Serum angiotensin-converting enzyme level is 127 U/L (normal: 19 to 95 U/L).

Which of the following is the most appropriate therapy for this patient?

(A) Prednisone
(B) Prednisone and melphalan
(C) Cyclophosphamide, hydroxydaunomycin (doxorubicin), Oncovin (vincristine), and prednisone (CHOP)
(D) Intravenous immune globulin

Item 47
A 56-year-old female smoker with poorly controlled hypercholesterolemia and the recent onset of crescendo angina was hospitalized for coronary artery bypass surgery after cardiac catheterization revealed triple vessel disease. There was no history of diabetes mellitus, hypertension, or renal disease. Her admission serum creatinine level was 0.9 mg/dL. Her operative course was marked by severe hypotension. Postoperatively, she continued to have hypotension without signs of congestive heart failure or fluid overload, and dopamine and volume resuscitation were started. The following day, blood cultures grew *Pseudomonas aeruginosa*, and gentamicin and ticarcillin were begun. Her serum creatinine level was 1.3 mg/dL.

On postoperative day 2, vasopressor therapy is continued. Her temperature is 37.0 °C (98.6 °F). Her pulse rate is 130/min, respiratory rate is 18/min, and blood pressure is 110/60 mm Hg. Bilateral crackles and an S_3 gallop are heard. Abdominal examination is normal. Sacral and 3+ peripheral edema are present. Neurologic examination shows that she is responsive but lethargic; there are no focal neurologic findings.

Laboratory studies:

Hemoglobin	10.0 g/dL
Hematocrit	31%
Leukocyte count	18,000/µL
Platelet count	456,000/µL
Blood urea nitrogen	36 mg/dL
Serum creatinine	2.3 mg/dL
Serum sodium	133 meq/L
Serum potassium	5.9 meq/L
Serum chloride	101 meq/L
Serum bicarbonate	17 meq/L

Urinalysis	Specific gravity 1.008; +1 protein, +1 blood, no glucose; 2–3 erythrocytes, 3 leukocytes/hpf, many granular casts

Urine output the previous 24 hours was 180 mL. Urine output does not increase appreciably after administration of 40 mg of furosemide and 5 mg of bumetanide over the next 4 hours.

Which of the following is most appropriate at this time?

(A) Perform renal biopsy
(B) Begin dialysis
(C) Obtain renal ultrasonography
(D) Discontinue aminoglycoside therapy and observe

Item 48
A 28-year-old man is brought to the emergency department because of a 4-day history of severe watery diarrhea, vomiting, and poor oral fluid intake. On physical examination, his temperature is 38.0 °C (100.4 °F). His pulse rate is 90/min seated and 124/min standing, and his blood pressure is 120/75 mm Hg seated and 80/50 mm Hg standing. A stool specimen is 1+ positive for occult blood. Examination is otherwise normal.

Laboratory studies:

Blood urea nitrogen	64 mg/dL
Serum creatinine	1.4 mg/dL
Serum sodium	142 meq/L
Serum potassium	3.4 meq/L
Serum chloride	106 meq/L
Serum bicarbonate	21 meq/L
Serum calcium	9.0 mg/dL
Urinalysis	Specific gravity 1.029, pH 5.5; 2–3 leukocytes/hpf; no casts

The elevated blood urea nitrogen:serum creatinine ratio is most likely due to which of the following mechanisms?

(A) Enhanced renal sodium, water, and urea reabsorption as a result of volume-mediated stimulation of antidiuretic hormone and renin-angiotensin-aldosterone
(B) Increased urea production as a result of gastrointestinal bleeding
(C) Shift of urea from the intracellular space to the extracellular space
(D) Fever

Item 49
A 22-year-old white woman is evaluated because of arthralgias, low-grade fever, malaise, and Raynaud's phenomenon. On physical examination, her temperature is 38.2 °C (100.8 °F), pulse rate is 94/min, and blood pressure is 145/92 mm Hg. A malar erythematous facial blush and livedo reticularis are present. Cardiac examination discloses a grade 2/6 systolic ejection murmur. The metacarpophalangeal and proximal interphalangeal joints are swollen, and there is 2+ bilateral ankle edema.

Laboratory studies:

Hematocrit	24%
Leukocyte count	2600/µL
Platelet count	102,000/µL
Blood urea nitrogen	36 mg/dL
Serum creatinine	2.4 mg/dL
Serum total complement	Reduced
Antinuclear antibody	Positive (1:640)
Anti-DNA antibody	Positive (1:840)
Urinalysis	4+ protein, 3+ heme; 8–15 erythrocytes/hpf, erythrocyte casts
24-Hour urinary protein	8 g/24 h

If a renal biopsy is performed, which of the following is most likely to be found?

(A) Membranous lupus nephropathy
(B) Mesangial lupus nephritis
(C) Focal proliferative lupus nephritis
(D) Diffuse proliferative lupus nephritis

Item 50
Which of the following is the most appropriate initial therapy for the patient in the preceding question?

(A) Monthly pulse intravenous methylprednisolone
(B) Oral glucocorticoids at high doses for at least 6 months
(C) Monthly pulse intravenous cyclophosphamide plus oral glucocorticoids
(D) Oral cyclosporine plus oral glucocorticoids

Item 51
A patient has the laboratory test results shown below:

Serum sodium	138 meq/L
Serum potassium	4.9 meq/L
Serum chloride	100 meq/L
Serum bicarbonate	15 meq/L

Arterial blood gas studies (patient breathing room air):

pH	7.48
P_{CO_2}	21 mm Hg
Bicarbonate	15 meq/L

Which of the following patients is most likely to have these acid-base parameters?

(A) A 2-year-old child who has accidentally swallowed an unknown quantity of his mother's aspirin
(B) A 28-year-old woman with bulimia and vomiting
(C) A 35-year-old man who has ingested a large amount of aspirin in a suicide attempt
(D) A 50-year-old woman with surreptitious laxative abuse

Item 52
A 34-year-old white male accountant is seen for a routine follow-up visit 2 years after undergoing cadaveric renal transplantation for end-stage renal disease secondary to glomerulonephritis. He states that he feels well except for occasional fatigue. He has had excellent allograft function on an immunosuppressive regimen of prednisone, 7.5 mg daily; cyclosporine, 125 mg twice daily; and azathioprine, 125 mg daily.

On physical examination, he looks well. Blood pressure is 158/88 mm Hg. The remainder of the examination is normal.

Laboratory studies:

Hemoglobin	17.9 g/dL
Hematocrit	56%
Leukocyte count	7450/µL; normal differential
Platelet count	218,000/µL
Serum creatinine	1.2 mg/dL
Serum cyclosporine	115 ng/mL (target: 100 to 225 ng/mL)

You note that his hematocrit has increased steadily from 43% to 56% over the past 6 to 9 months and order measurement of erythrocyte mass and plasma volume. The erythrocyte mass is reported to be elevated, and the plasma volume is normal.

After initial phlebotomy, which of the following long-term therapeutic options is most appropriate?

(A) Change azathioprine to mycophenolate
(B) Begin an angiotensin-converting enzyme inhibitor
(C) Change cyclosporine to tacrolimus
(D) Begin melphalan

Item 53
A 72-year-old man is brought to the emergency department because of anorexia, disorientation, and lassitude. He has been in good health since a motor vehicle accident 12 years earlier, which necessitated extensive abdominal surgery. There is no history of diabetes mellitus, hypertension, or renal disease. He last saw a physician 6 years ago.

On physical examination, his pulse rate is 118/min and regular, and blood pressure is 170/100 mm Hg without orthostatic changes. There is moderate neck vein distention. Bilateral crackles are audible, and an S_3 gallop is heard at the left sternal border. His abdomen is nontender, no bruit is heard, and there are no enlarged abdominal organs. Popliteal and pedal pulses are normal. There is no discoloration of his toes or pedal edema. The patient is somnolent but oriented.

Laboratory studies:

Hematocrit	32%
Mean corpuscular volume	Normal
Leukocyte count	5500/µL
Platelet count	199,000/µL
Blood urea nitrogen	113 mg/dL
Serum creatinine	8.7 mg/dL
Serum sodium	139 meq/L
Serum potassium	5.6 meq/L
Serum chloride	98 meq/L
Serum bicarbonate	18 meq/L
Urinalysis	Specific gravity 1.011; trace protein, no blood, glucose, or ketones; normal microscopic examination
Urinary sodium	47 meq/L

Renal ultrasonography shows normal-sized kidneys and no evidence of hydronephrosis. Urine output over the first 12 hours of hospitalization is 480 mL.

Which of the following is the most appropriate first step in managing this patient?

(A) Obtain CT of the kidneys and pelvis without contrast
(B) Administer volume repletion
(C) Obtain emergent renal arteriography
(D) Administer pulse intravenous glucocorticoids
(E) Enroll the patient in chronic end-stage renal disease hemodialysis program after obtaining informed consent

Item 54
A 60-year-old man has chronic obstructive pulmonary disease and congestive heart failure. Current medications are digoxin, theophylline, loop diuretics, angiotensin-converting enzyme inhibitors, and spironolactone. He is hospitalized because of an exacerbation of his lung disease caused by an intercurrent infection. His clinical condition deteriorates, and endotracheal intubation and mechanical ventilation are required.

After 1 week, he has improved, but the pulmonologists are having difficulty weaning him from the ventilator. He is currently receiving furosemide, 80 mg every 8 hours, to maintain diuresis. Physical examination shows bilateral crackles and 2+ peripheral edema.

Laboratory studies:

Blood urea nitrogen	52 mg/dL
Serum creatinine	2.1 mg/dL
Serum sodium	131 meq/L
Serum potassium	5.5 meq/L
Serum chloride	80 meq/L
Serum bicarbonate	38 meq/L

Arterial blood gas studies (patient on the ventilator):

pH	7.48
P_{CO_2}	50 mm Hg
Bicarbonate	36 meq/L

Which of the following would be most helpful in weaning this patient from the ventilator?

(A) Continue aggressive diuresis with loop diuretics
(B) Discontinue all diuretics and begin normal saline, 100 mL/h
(C) Change furosemide to acetazolamide
(D) Begin continuous arteriovenous ultrafiltration

Item 55
A 61-year-old female teacher requests a second opinion regarding her recently diagnosed "white coat" hypertension. For the past 4 months, her blood pressure readings (measured in the office by both her primary care physician and his nurse) have averaged 165/90 mm Hg. However, repeated blood pressure measurements that she obtains at home average 130/76 mm Hg. She requests your opinion about the diagnosis and her risk for cardiovascular disease.

Which of the following statements is correct?

(A) The risk of hypertensive cardiovascular complications (including left ventricular hypertrophy) correlates more closely with office blood pressure readings than with 24-hour or daytime ambulatory blood pressure readings
(B) Physicians should routinely measure the office blood pressure of their patients because readings obtained by physicians are lower than those obtained by nurses
(C) Since "white coat" hypertension may affect almost 20% of patients with mild office hypertension, all patients with this suspected diagnosis should undergo ambulatory blood pressure monitoring with an automated device
(D) Patients with "white coat" hypertension have a higher systemic vascular resistance and left ventricular mass index than their normotensive counterparts and may have an increased risk of cardiovascular disease

Item 56
A 36-year-old obese pregnant woman is referred for evaluation. She has four healthy children following uncomplicated term pregnancies. She has had hypertension for 5 years that is currently well controlled with ramipril. There is also a family history of hypertension. She was first seen for prenatal care by a physician 2 months after her last menstrual period. Her pregnancy had been uneventful, and she had gained 2.7 kg (6 lb). Her blood pressure was 140/92 mm Hg, and she had trace edema.

Laboratory studies:

Hematocrit	33%
Blood urea nitrogen	11 mg/dL
Serum creatinine	0.7 mg/dL
Serum uric acid	4.1 mg/dL
Urinalysis	Trace protein
Urinary protein	125 mg/24 h
Creatinine clearance	160 mL/min

Which of the following statements is not correct regarding this patient?

(A) Her ramipril should be discontinued
(B) She should be started on another antihypertensive agent
(C) She should be told that she has an approximately 25% risk of developing preeclampsia
(D) She should be told that better control of blood pressure will diminish her risk of developing preeclampsia

Item 57
An otherwise healthy 41-year-old man has had recurrent calcium oxalate nephrolithiasis for the past 3 years. A recent 24-hour urine collection showed the following:

Creatinine	1.56 g/24 h
Calcium	380 mg/24 h
Urate	740 mg/24 h (normal: < 750 mg/24 h)
Oxalate	38 mg/24 h (normal: < 40 mg/24 h)
Citrate	643 mg/24 h (normal: 300 to 700 mg/24 h)
Sodium	104 meq/24 h

Which of the following would be most effective in reducing his urinary calcium excretion?

(A) Dietary calcium restriction
(B) Cranberry juice
(C) Hydrochlorothiazide
(D) Furosemide
(E) High fluid intake

Item 58
Which of the following genetic renal disorders is usually associated with renal failure?

(A) Medullary sponge kidney
(B) Nephrogenic diabetes insipidus
(C) Thin basement membrane disease
(D) Nephronophthisis and medullary cystic disease

Item 59
A 28-year-old woman with cystic fibrosis was hospitalized 2 weeks ago because of fever, cough, purulent yellow-green sputum, and a new right lower lobe infiltrate. She has been treated with tobramycin and piperacillin intravenously since admission. Her renal function, which was normal on admission, has deteriorated. Her blood urea nitrogen level has increased from 14 mg/dL to 32 mg/dL, and her serum creatinine concentration has risen from 0.6 mg/dL to 3.2 mg/dL. There has been no decrease in urine output during this period. Additional medications have included ibuprofen for chest discomfort.

On physical examination, her temperature is 38.3 °C (101.0 °F). Her pulse rate is 88/min, respiratory rate is 14/min and unlabored, and blood pressure is 130/72 mm Hg. There is a faint blanching maculopapular rash on her trunk and upper extremities. Examination of her chest shows only scattered rhonchi. The remainder of the examination is normal.

Laboratory studies:

Hematocrit	38%
Leukocyte count	7500/µL
Platelet count	325,000/µL
Blood urea nitrogen	32 mg/dL
Serum creatinine	3.2 mg/dL
Serum electrolytes	Normal
Urinalysis	Trace protein, 4+ heme; many leukocytes and erythrocytes/hpf, no erythrocyte casts

Chest radiograph confirms that the pulmonary infiltrate is resolving.

Which of the following is the most appropriate diagnostic study at this time?

(A) Intravenous pyelography
(B) Wright or Hansel stain of the urine sediment
(C) Determination of serum tobramycin level
(D) 24-Hour urine for calcium and oxalate

Item 60
A 23-year-old man is evaluated because of increasing dyspnea. He has a history of intravenous drug use and known HIV infection. Chest radiograph shows bilateral infiltrates. The patient is hospitalized. His blood pressure on admission is 120/76 mm Hg.

Laboratory studies on admission:

Blood urea nitrogen	20 mg/dL
Serum creatinine	1.3 mg/dL
Serum sodium	131 meq/L
Serum potassium	4.8 meq/L
Serum chloride	95 meq/L
Serum bicarbonate	22 meq/L

Further evaluation leads to a diagnosis of *Pneumocystis carinii* pneumonia, and parenteral trimethoprim-sulfamethoxazole is begun.

Laboratory studies one week after admission:

Blood urea nitrogen	25 mg/dL
Serum creatinine	1.8 mg/dL
Serum sodium	130 meq/L
Serum potassium	6.2 meq/L
Serum chloride	93 meq/L
Serum bicarbonate	24 meq/L

Which of the following is the most likely cause of the increased potassium concentration in this patient?

(A) Lung tissue destruction due to *P. carinii* infection
(B) Decreased renal potassium excretion due to deteriorating renal function
(C) Blockade of distal renal tubule potassium excretion due to trimethoprim
(D) Interstitial nephritis due to sulfamethoxazole
(E) Addison's disease due to adrenal HIV infection

Item 61
A 48-year-old white man is evaluated because of cough, arthralgias, malaise, and weight loss. He had a normal annual physical examination and renal function studies 2 months ago.

On physical examination today, his temperature is 37.3 °C (99.2 °F). His pulse rate is 92/min and regular, respiratory rate is 24/min, and blood pressure is 160/94 mm Hg. Cardiac examination is normal. Examination of the chest discloses crackles and rhonchi at the left base. Examination of the abdomen and extremities is normal.

Laboratory studies:

Hematocrit	34%
Leukocyte count	12,000/µL
Platelet count	425,000/µL
Plasma glucose	Normal
Blood urea nitrogen	25 mg/dL

Serum creatinine	1.8 mg/dL
Serum electrolytes	Normal
Urinalysis	3+ protein, 4+ heme; many erythrocytes/hpf, many dysmorphic erythrocytes
24-Hour urinary protein	2.7 g/24 h

A chest radiograph shows a hazy left lower lobe infiltrate. An electrocardiogram is normal. Renal ultrasonography shows normal kidney size and texture.

Which of the following diagnostic studies should be done next?

(A) Determinations of serum HIV antibodies and HIV viral load
(B) Antineutrophil cytoplasmic antibody (ANCA) and anti–glomerular basement membrane (anti-GBM) antibody assays
(C) Serum and urine protein electrophoresis
(D) Serologic tests for hepatitis B and C

Item 62

A renal biopsy is performed on the patient in the preceding question. The biopsy specimen shows focal and segmental necrotizing glomerulonephritis with crescent formation. Immunofluorescence shows no immune staining.

Which of the following is the most appropriate initial therapy?

(A) Cyclophosphamide and glucocorticoids
(B) Cyclophosphamide, glucocorticoids, and plasmapheresis
(C) Cyclosporine and glucocorticoids
(D) Cyclosporine, glucocorticoids, and plasmapheresis

Item 63

A 56-year-old white woman requests a second opinion regarding her primary care physician's diagnosis of "microprotein in my urine" 1 month ago. She has a 6-year history of type 2 diabetes mellitus and hypertension. Medical history is otherwise unremarkable. Medications include glipizide, 5 mg each morning; sustained-release nifedipine, 30 mg daily; and daily aspirin. She follows an American Diabetes Association diet.

On physical examination, the patient appears well. She weighs 47 kg (103 lb). Blood pressure is 148/92 mm Hg seated and standing. Funduscopic examination shows background diabetic retinopathy without hemorrhages, exudates, or papilledema. There is no peripheral edema. The remainder of the examination is normal.

Laboratory studies:

Complete blood count	Normal
Hemoglobin A_{1C}	6.3% (normal: 4.0% to 6.0%)
Plasma glucose (fasting)	121 mg/dL
Blood urea nitrogen	Normal
Serum creatinine	Normal
Serum electrolytes	Normal
Serum thyroid-stimulating hormone	Normal
Urinalysis	Routine urinalysis normal; microalbumin assay of the albumin:creatinine ratio 50 mg/g

The patient requests your opinion regarding her diagnosis of microalbuminuria and its implications regarding her therapy and risks for renal disease.

Which of the following statements is correct?

(A) The presence of microalbuminuria in a patient with type 1 or type 2 diabetes mellitus is usually indicative of early diabetic nephropathy
(B) Almost all patients with type 2 diabetes mellitus who have microalbuminuria develop overt nephropathy over a 10-year-period
(C) For patients with type 2 diabetes mellitus and essential hypertension, the risk of cardiovascular disease is not influenced by the presence of microalbuminuria
(D) Optimal therapy for diabetic patients with microalbuminuria who are taking nifedipine is to increase the nifedipine dose to optimize control of blood pressure

Item 64

A 28-year-old man is found to have microscopic hematuria on an insurance physical examination. His physical examination in your office is normal. Complete blood count, plasma glucose, blood urea nitrogen, serum creatinine, and serum electrolytes are normal. Urinalysis shows no protein, many erythrocytes/hpf, no erythrocyte casts, and no dysmorphic erythrocytes. Urine culture shows no growth, and an intravenous pyelogram is reported as showing medullary sponge kidney but no stones or other abnormalities.

Appropriate counseling of this patient includes which of the following?

(A) Advise him that this disorder is likely to progress to chronic renal failure over 10 to 20 years
(B) Advise him that this is a benign finding and that although it may be a risk factor for nephrolithiasis, it never leads to progressive renal failure
(C) Advise him to have his children undergo genetic testing for this disorder so that they can be treated appropriately at an early age
(D) Advise him that the course of this disorder can be modified by treatment with an angiotensin-converting enzyme inhibitor

Item 65

A 31-year-old woman is evaluated 2 days after she passed a kidney stone following 3 days of left-sided renal colic. She has a 10-year history of recurrent episodes of calcium phosphate nephrolithiasis. At age 17, she developed inflammatory bowel disease. For the past 2 years, she has had symptoms of dry eyes, dry mouth, and Raynaud's phenomenon.

Laboratory studies:

Blood urea nitrogen	15 mg/dL
Serum creatinine	1.2 mg/dL
Serum sodium	142 meq/L
Serum potassium	2.9 meq/L
Serum chloride	112 meq/L
Serum bicarbonate	20 meq/L
Urinalysis	Specific gravity 1.015, pH 6.5, 2+ heme, no protein, 3–10 erythrocytes/hpf

A plain radiograph of the abdomen and pelvis shows multiple 1- to 2-mm calcifications overlying both renal shadows.

Which of the following is the most likely cause of the renal stone disease in this patient?

(A) Idiopathic hypercalciuria
(B) Cystinuria
(C) Renal tubular acidosis
(D) Struvite (infection) stone disease
(E) Medullary sponge kidney

Item 66
A 65-year-old man is seen for a routine annual evaluation. He states that he has been feeling fatigued and exhausted. He is normotensive, and his physical examination is normal.

Laboratory studies:

Hematocrit	25%
Leukocyte count	5600/µL
Platelet count	340,000/µL
Plasma glucose	78 mg/dL
Blood urea nitrogen	28 mg/dL
Serum creatinine	2.1 mg/dL
Serum sodium	135 meq/L
Serum potassium	5.0 meq/L
Serum chloride	105 meq/L
Serum bicarbonate	28 meq/L
Serum calcium	10.9 mg/dL
Serum phosphorus	4.9 mg/dL
Urinalysis	Trace protein; normal sediment
Creatinine clearance	48 mL/min
24-Hour urinary protein	2.8 g/24 h

Which of the following is the most appropriate diagnostic test at this time?

(A) Intravenous pyelography
(B) Urine immunoelectrophoresis
(C) Serum angiotensin-converting enzyme determination
(D) Serum complement determination and antinuclear antibody assay

Item 67
A 30-year-old man has a history of a seizure disorder following head trauma 5 years ago. Treatment with phenytoin has controlled his seizures adequately. He has a grand mal seizure while "partying" late one evening and is brought to the emergency department by his friends. The friends state that they had all been drinking alcohol but deny use of any illicit drugs or stimulants.

On physical examination, the patient is a well-developed, muscular young man who is very lethargic and confused. He is afebrile. His pulse rate is 100/min and regular, respiratory rate is 18/min and deep, and blood pressure is 130/95 mm Hg. Examination is unremarkable except for the lethargy and confusion.

Laboratory studies:

Complete blood count	Normal
Blood urea nitrogen	12 mg/dL
Serum creatinine	1.0 mg/dL
Serum sodium	140 meq/L
Serum potassium	4.8 meq/L
Serum chloride	100 meq/L
Serum bicarbonate	12 meq/L
Serum osmolality (measured)	310 mosm/L
Arterial blood gas studies (patient breathing room air):	
pH	7.25
Pco_2	28 mm Hg
Bicarbonate (calculated)	12 meq/L
Blood ethanol	100 mg/dL
Urinalysis	Normal

Which of the following is the most appropriate initial treatment for the metabolic acidosis and osmotic gap in this patient?

(A) Observation and repeat arterial blood gas studies in 2 hours
(B) Sodium bicarbonate, 2 ampules (100 meq) by intravenous push
(C) One liter of 5% dextrose in water plus bicarbonate, 3 ampules (150 meq), infused over 3 hours
(D) Hemodialysis
(E) Fomepizole

Item 68

A 23-year-old female graduate student requests a second opinion because of "microalbuminuria and normal blood pressure." The patient has had type 1 diabetes mellitus for 9 years managed with diet, exercise, and split-dose insulin therapy. She states that she carefully adheres to her diabetes regimen. Her primary care physician noted microalbuminuria during routine screening last month. She denies other target organ damage due to diabetes. Blood pressure determinations both in the office and at home average 130/85 mm Hg.

On physical examination, she appears well. Her weight is 62 kg (136 lb). Blood pressure is 128/82 mm Hg seated and standing. Examination is normal.

The following laboratory studies are normal: complete blood count, plasma glucose, blood urea nitrogen, serum creatinine, and serum electrolytes. Hemoglobin A_{1C} is 5.8% (normal: 4.0% to 6.0%). Routine urinalysis is normal.

The patient's primary care physician wants to begin antihypertensive therapy for her recently discovered microalbuminuria. She is very concerned about the possibility of developing renal disease, but also is concerned about the advisability of taking antihypertensive drugs, since her blood pressure is normal.

Which of the following statements is correct?

(A) Progression to overt nephropathy occurs in greater than 70% of patients with type 1 diabetes mellitus and microalbuminuria, especially if microalbuminuria develops more than 15 years following the diagnosis of diabetes mellitus
(B) Therapy with an angiotensin-converting enzyme (ACE) inhibitor is likely to reduce the degree of microalbuminuria and significantly lessen the chance of progression to overt nephropathy in patients with type 1 diabetes mellitus and microalbuminuria
(C) The risk of developing microalbuminuria does not correlate with glycemic control, and strict glycemic control does not reduce the risk of developing microalbuminuria
(D) Therapy with an ACE inhibitor has been proved to lessen the chance of developing overt nephropathy in all patients with type 1 diabetes mellitus, even patients who do not have hypertension or microalbuminuria

Item 69

A 38-year-old woman with biopsy-proven focal segmental glomerulosclerosis has a serum creatinine level of 2.0 mg/dL, a 24-hour creatinine clearance of 48 mL/min, and a 24-hour urinary protein excretion of 3.7 g. Her glomerular filtration rate (GFR), using iothalamate as a marker (true GFR), is 32 mL/min.

Which of the following mechanisms explains why the creatinine clearance overestimates the true GFR in this patient?

(A) Increased tubular secretion of creatinine
(B) Decreased reabsorption of filtered creatinine
(C) Increased release of creatinine from muscle
(D) Decreased tubular secretion of creatinine

Item 70

A 55-year-old man is evaluated because of a 10-day history of a severe sore throat. One year ago, he had a soft tissue sarcoma of his right thumb, leading to surgical amputation, radiation therapy to his right axilla, and chemotherapy with carboplatin and ifosfamide. At that time, extensive evaluation revealed no metastases and normal renal function.

On physical examination, his temperature is 37.2 °C (99.0 °F). His pulse rate is 88/min and regular, respiratory rate is 14/min, and blood pressure is 130/86 mm Hg. The right thumb is absent. Examination is otherwise normal.

Laboratory studies:

Complete blood count	Normal
Plasma glucose	Normal
Blood urea nitrogen	42 mg/dL
Serum creatinine	3.8 mg/dL
Serum electrolytes	Normal
Urinalysis	No protein; 2–5 leukocytes, 2–5 erythrocytes/hpf

Renal ultrasonography shows no hydronephrosis.

Which of the following is the most likely diagnosis?

(A) Poststreptococcal glomerulonephritis
(B) IgA nephropathy
(C) Radiation nephritis
(D) Ifosfamide interstitial nephritis

Item 71

A 39-year-old male computer analyst with a 6-year history of autosomal dominant polycystic kidney disease (ADPKD) is evaluated because of intermittent left flank pain. He does not have fever, chills, dysuria, or a history of trauma. Since being diagnosed with ADPKD, he has not had urinary tract infections, hematuria, or renal calculi. Over the past 4 years, his serum creatinine level has slowly risen from 1.4 mg/dL to 1.9 mg/dL (at the time of his last visit 4 weeks ago). Lisinopril, 10 mg daily, was started 2 years ago for management of stage 1 hypertension (blood pressure 158/92 mm Hg). He has not taken nonsteroidal anti-inflammatory drugs recently and has not been exposed to contrast agents or any other nephrotoxins.

On physical examination, his blood pressure is 138/88 mm Hg seated and standing. Examination of the head and neck and cardiopulmonary examination are normal. Polycystic kidneys are easily palpated bilaterally, and there is mild tenderness in the left flank. Neuromuscular examination is normal. There is no peripheral edema.

Laboratory studies:

Complete blood count	Normal
Blood urea nitrogen	43 mg/dL
Serum creatinine	4.2 mg/dL

Serum sodium	138 meq/L
Serum potassium	5.3 meq/L
Serum chloride	100 meq/L
Serum bicarbonate	22 meq/L
Serum calcium	9.2 mg/dL
Serum phosphorus	4.2 mg/dL
Serum uric acid	8.2 mg/dL
Urinalysis	Trace protein, 2+ heme, no glucose; 0–2 leukocytes, 10–15 erythrocytes/hpf, no casts

A plain radiograph of the abdomen and pelvis is normal. There are no calcifications or radiopaque densities over the left renal bed, ureteral tract, or bladder. CT of the abdomen without contrast shows 15-cm kidneys bilaterally with innumerable cysts but no hemorrhage. There is a 5-mm density at the left ureteropelvic junction with some hydronephrosis of the collecting system.

Which of the following is the most likely explanation for this patient's findings?

(A) Natural progression of ADPKD
(B) Complication of angiotensin-converting enzyme inhibitor therapy
(C) Renal calculus
(D) Hemorrhage or infection of a cyst

Item 72
A 60-year-old man is evaluated because of 1-month history of headache and palpitations. The patient has progressive renal insufficiency secondary to chronic glomerulonephritis. He also has had chronic obstructive pulmonary disease for 10 years, treated with inhaled bronchodilators and glucocorticoids. There is no history of hypertension. Medications include prednisone, 10 mg daily; ferrous sulfate, 325 mg daily; albuterol, 2 puffs 4 times daily; and ipratropium bromide, 2 puffs 3 times daily. He has also received erythropoietin, 10,000 units subcutaneously once a week, for the past 2 months for the anemia associated with his renal insufficiency. His blood pressure 2 months ago was 130/80 mm Hg, hematocrit was 27%, and serum creatinine was 3.5 mg/dL.

On physical examination, the patient appears alert and comfortable. He weighs 97 kg (213 lb). Temperature is 36.6 °C (98.0 °F). His pulse rate is 90/min, and blood pressure is 160/110 mm Hg. There is no neck vein distention. The lung fields are clear, and cardiac examination is normal. His abdomen is obese without palpable tenderness or enlarged organs. There is trace pedal edema bilaterally.

Laboratory studies:

Hemoglobin	12.0 g/dL
Hematocrit	36%
Leukocyte count	6500/µL
Platelet count	260,000/µL
Blood urea nitrogen	57 mg/dL
Serum creatinine	3.7 mg/dL
Serum sodium	135 meq/L
Serum potassium	3.9 meq/L
Serum chloride	100 meq/L
Serum bicarbonate	20 meq/L

Which of the following best explains this patient's new-onset hypertension?

(A) Essential hypertension
(B) Worsening renal failure with fluid retention
(C) Complication of erythropoietin administration
(D) Iatrogenic Cushing's syndrome

Item 73
A 42-year-old woman with known sickle cell disease and longstanding nocturia and polyuria is evaluated because of new-onset painless gross hematuria. On physical examination, her temperature is 37.1 °C (98.8 °F). Her pulse rate is 110/min and regular, respiratory rate is 14/min, and blood pressure is 135/86 mm Hg. Cardiac examination shows a grade 2/6 systolic ejection murmur. The remainder of the physical examination is normal.

Laboratory studies:

Hematocrit	27%
Leukocyte count	5000/µL
Platelet count	320,000/µL
Plasma glucose	Normal
Blood urea nitrogen	Normal
Serum creatinine	Normal
Serum electrolytes	Normal
Urinalysis	Many erythrocytes/hpf, no erythrocyte casts
Urine culture	No growth

Which of the following diagnostic studies is most appropriate at this time?

(A) Ultrasonography of the kidneys
(B) CT of the kidneys
(C) CT of the kidneys and cystoscopy
(D) Renal angiography

Item 74
A 39-year-old man is brought to the emergency department because of a 12-hour history of abdominal pain and nausea. He has chronic focal and segmental glomerulo-

sclerosis with a baseline serum creatinine concentration of 2.1 mg/dL and a urinary protein excretion of 2 g/24 h. A serum creatinine determination in the emergency department is 2.0 mg/dL, and CT of the abdomen with contrast is normal. Thirty hours later, his serum creatinine is 3.2 mg/dL, and urine output has fallen to 20 mL/h. Because of the acute renal failure, you suspect a diagnosis of contrast-induced acute tubular necrosis.

Which of the following urinalysis findings is most compatible with your diagnosis?

(A)

Specific Gravity	Protein	Blood	Microscopic Examination
1.012	2+	2+	20–30 erythrocytes, 15–20 leukocytes/hpf; Hansel's stain positive for eosinophils (< 5% leukocytes)

(B)

1.010	2+	Negative	1–3 leukocytes, 5–10 renal tubular cells/hpf; many pigmented granular casts, occasional renal tubular cell casts; Hansel's stain negative

(C)

1.012	2+	2+	5–10 erythrocytes , 25–50 leukocytes/hpf; many bacteria, occasional finely granular casts; Hansel's stain negative

(D)

1.020	2+	2+ to 3+	10–20 erythrocytes, 2–4 leukocytes/hpf; 1–3 erythrocyte casts/hpf; Hansel's stain negative

Item 75

A 55-year-old white woman with chronic low back pain and chronic polyuria and nocturia is found to have renal dysfunction during a routine annual evaluation. She has no significant medical history and does not use any medications. Physical examination is normal.

Laboratory studies:

Complete blood count	Normal
Plasma glucose	Normal
Blood urea nitrogen	28 mg/dL
Serum creatinine	2.3 mg/dL
Serum electrolytes	Normal
Urinalysis	No protein; no erythrocytes, 5–10 leukocytes/hpf, no casts
Urine culture	No growth

Renal ultrasonography suggests normal-sized kidneys without hydronephrosis but with papillary necrosis.

Which of the following should be done next?

(A) Screen the patient for hemoglobin SA trait
(B) Perform a glucose tolerance test
(C) Obtain a urine culture for *Mycobacterium tuberculosis*
(D) Ask the patient again about use of prescribed drugs and over-the-counter medications

Item 76

A 30-year-old woman has a long history of Crohn's disease. She has required multiple abdominal procedures and has an ileostomy. She usually controls her ostomy output with loperamide. For the past week, she has noted increased ostomy output, weakness, and paresthesias. She comes to the emergency department and is subsequently hospitalized.

Physical examination on admission discloses that her blood pressure is 115/75 mm Hg supine and 105/65 mm Hg seated. Her skin is normal. Cardiopulmonary examination is normal. Her abdomen is not tender. She has multiple surgical scars and a functioning ileostomy. There is 1+ peripheral edema.

Laboratory studies on admission:

Blood urea nitrogen	30 mg/dL
Serum creatinine	2.0 mg/dL
Serum sodium	129 meq/L
Serum potassium	2.9 meq/L
Serum chloride	85 meq/L
Serum bicarbonate	18 meq/L
Serum calcium	5.5 mg/dL
Serum phosphorus	1.3 mg/dL
Serum albumin	3.2 g/dL

Intravenous fluids consisting of alternating bags of isotonic saline plus 40 meq/L of potassium chloride and half-normal isotonic saline plus 40 meq/L of potassium chloride and 50 meq/L of sodium bicarbonate are begun at 150 mL/h. After 24 hours, the orthostatic changes are reversed. Her blood urea nitrogen level has fallen to 20 mg/dL, and her serum creatinine concentration has decreased to 1.5 mg/dL. Serum bicarbonate concentration is 22 meq/L. However, her serum potassium level is still 2.9 meq/L, and her serum calcium level is 5.3 mg/dL.

Which of the following is the most likely reason for the persistent hypokalemia?

(A) The patient is likely magnesium depleted, which prevents potassium repletion
(B) The persistent hypocalcemia makes correction of hypokalemia more difficult
(C) The administered sodium bicarbonate is shifting potassium into cells
(D) The hypophosphatemia has exacerbated the hypokalemia

Item 77
A 63-year-old woman with diabetic nephropathy comes to your office for a routine visit after returning from a Caribbean cruise. She has a 20-year history of hypertension and type 2 diabetes mellitus. Medications include lisinopril, 10 mg daily, and a calcium supplement. The patient is concerned about her diabetes mellitus and kidney disease because of "dietary indiscretions" on the cruise ship.

On physical examination, her pulse rate is 90/min, and blood pressure is 150/92 mm Hg. Funduscopic examination shows hypertensive diabetic retinopathy. Cardiopulmonary and abdominal examinations are normal. There are no neuromuscular deficits, but 2+ bilateral pedal edema is noted.

Laboratory studies:

Hematocrit	28%
Blood urea nitrogen	54 mg/dL
Serum creatinine	4.9 mg/dL (stable value)
Serum calcium	8.8 mg/dL
Serum phosphorus	7.5 mg/dL
Serum uric acid	10.9 mg/dL
Serum albumin	2.9 g/dL
Serum parathyroid hormone	258 pg/mL (normal: < 50 pg/mL)
Serum protein electrophoresis	Normal
Urine protein electrophoresis	Normal

In addition to recommending a low-phosphorus diet, which of the following is the most appropriate initial therapy for this patient's hyperphosphatemia?

(A) Calcium-containing phosphate binders with meals
(B) 1,25-Dihydroxyvitamin D (Rocaltrol) each morning
(C) Aluminum hydroxide with meals
(D) Magnesium hydroxide with meals

Item 78
An 18-year-old man becomes despondent after an argument with his girlfriend. He swallows a "poison" and 3 hours later comes to the emergency department. He states that he threw the bottle into a sewer, and it cannot be recovered. He is not aware of the specific chemical that he ingested, but knows only that the bottle had a skull and crossbones on the label.

The patient is disheveled and anxious. Physical examination is otherwise normal.

Laboratory studies:

Blood urea nitrogen	30 mg/dL
Serum creatinine	1.8 mg/dL
Serum sodium	140 meq/L
Serum potassium	5.3 meq/L
Serum chloride	100 meq/L
Serum bicarbonate	10 meq/L
Arterial blood gas studies (patient breathing room air):	
pH	7.16
P_{CO_2}	23 mm Hg
P_{O_2}	100 mm Hg
Bicarbonate	8 meq/L
Urinalysis	Many erythrocytes/hpf, many rectangular crystals

Which of the following poisons did this patient most likely ingest?

(A) Ethylene glycol
(B) Methanol
(C) Isopropyl alcohol
(D) Cyanide
(E) Calcium oxalate

Item 79
A 50-year-old woman is evaluated because of "spells" characterized by throbbing headache, hypertension, chest discomfort with palpitations, nausea, dizziness, and sweating. These episodes have occurred periodically throughout her life, but both the frequency and the intensity have increased recently. She also reports a history of high blood pressure, and her former primary care physician had tried multiple combinations of medications with only moderate success. Current medications include an estradiol patch, 0.25 mg daily; felodipine, 10 mg daily; labetalol, 300 mg twice daily; hydrochlorothiazide, 25 mg daily; and aspirin, 81 mg daily.

On physical examination, the patient is thin and anxious but is in no acute distress. Her weight is 54.2 kg (119 lb). Her pulse rate is 90/min, respiratory rate is 18/min, and blood pressure is 189/99 mm Hg supine and 154/84 mm Hg standing. The remainder of the physical examination is normal.

Laboratory studies:

Complete blood count	Normal
Plasma glucose (fasting)	125 mg/dL
Blood urea nitrogen	14 mg/dL
Serum creatinine	0.9 mg/dL
Serum sodium	142 meq/L
Serum potassium	4.3 meq/L
Serum chloride	100 meq/L
Serum bicarbonate	28 meq/L
Serum thyroid function studies	Normal

Plasma norepinephrine	1156 pg/mL (normal: 100 to 450 pg/mL)
Urinary norepinephrine	1270 nmol/24 h (normal: 590 to 855 nmol/24 h)
Urinary epinephrine	273 nmol/24 h (normal: < 275 nmol/24 h)
Urinary vanillylmandelic acid	32 µmol/24 h (normal: < 35 µmol/24 h)
Urinary creatinine	15 mg/kg/24 h

Which of the following statements is correct regarding this patient?

(A) The elevated plasma and urinary catecholamine levels are diagnostic for pheochromocytoma, and the patient should undergo laparoscopic adrenalectomy
(B) An elevated plasma glucose level is found only when a pheochromocytoma is associated with one of the multiple endocrine neoplasia (MEN) syndromes
(C) This patient's antihypertensive medications may increase norepinephrine levels, and the test should be repeated after proper adjustments of medications
(D) The diagnosis of pheochromocytoma is best approached by bilateral adrenal vein sampling for metanephrine
(E) Pheochromocytoma is unlikely in this age group and is not associated with orthostatic changes in blood pressure

Items 80, 81
A 23-year-old pregnant woman was seen by her obstetrician 2 months after her last menstrual period. This is her first pregnancy, and she has had no personal or family history of diabetes mellitus, renal disease, or hypertension. On physical examination, her pulse rate was 82/min, and her blood pressure was 90/60 mm Hg. Her serum creatinine concentration was 0.4 mg/dL. Over the next 2 months, she was continually troubled by vomiting. Her ability to eat was severely limited, and she only gained 0.9 kg (2 lb).

At her 4-month visit, her pulse rate is 110/min seated and 130/min standing, and her blood pressure is 83/60 mm Hg seated and 60 mm Hg systolic standing. There is no jugular venous distention. Her chest is clear, and there is no murmur, gallop, or rub. Her abdomen is nontender. Pelvic examination shows a 16-week gravid uterus. She has no pedal edema. Neurologic examination is normal.

Laboratory studies:

Hematocrit	32%
Leukocyte count	5300/µL
Platelet count	299,000/µL
Blood urea nitrogen	26 mg/dL
Serum creatinine	1.3 mg/dL
Peripheral blood smear	Microcytic erythrocytes
Urinalysis	Specific gravity 1.020; trace protein, no blood, ketones, or glucose; normal microscopic examination

Item 80
Which of the following is the most likely cause of this patient's renal insufficiency?

(A) Preeclampsia
(B) Vomiting
(C) Thrombotic microangiopathy
(D) Urinary tract obstruction
(E) Systemic lupus erythematosus

Item 81
Which of the following is the most appropriate treatment for the patient in the preceding question?

(A) Volume repletion with normal saline and provision of nutrition
(B) Plasmapheresis
(C) Therapeutic abortion
(D) Glucocorticoids

Item 82
In which of the following clinical situations would an increase in the serum creatinine concentration be explained only by a reduction in the glomerular filtration rate?

(A) Use of trimethoprim in a patient with a urinary tract infection
(B) Increased levels of ketoacids in a patient with diabetic acidosis
(C) Severe extracellular volume contraction in a patient with diarrhea
(D) Use of cimetidine in a patient with a peptic ulcer
(E) Seizures in a patient with status epilepticus

Item 83
A 48-year-old businessman is brought to the emergency department because of substernal chest pain and weakness. An acute myocardial infarction is diagnosed, and he is transferred to the cardiac care unit. He has a 5-year history of hypertension and has been treated with hydrochlorothiazide with an excellent response. The patient smokes one pack of cigarettes a day and drinks about two alcoholic beverages daily.

On physical examination in the cardiac care unit, his pulse rate is 80/min and regular, and his blood pressure is 126/80 mm Hg without orthostatic changes. There is no neck vein distention or edema. Cardiac and abdominal examinations are normal.

Laboratory studies:

Blood urea nitrogen	12 mg/dL
Serum creatinine	1.0 mg/dL
Serum sodium	137 meq/L
Serum potassium	3.1 meq/L
Serum chloride	99 meq/L
Serum bicarbonate	28 meq/L
Serum calcium	7.8 mg/dL
Serum magnesium	0.7 mg/dL
Urinalysis	Specific gravity 1.013; trace protein, no ketones or glucose; normal microscopic examination

An electrocardiogram shows normal sinus rhythm, ST elevations in the inferior leads, and peaked T waves across the precordial leads.

Which of the following is the most appropriate first step in correcting the electrolyte disorder in this patient?

(A) Discontinue hydrochlorothiazide
(B) Administer magnesium sulfate intravenously
(C) Administer calcium gluconate intravenously
(D) Administer volume repletion

Index — Nephrology

Note: Page numbers followed by *f* indicate illustrations; those followed by *t* indicate tables.